T0358996

Thoracic Surgery in the Special Care Patient

Editor

SHARON BEN-OR

THORACIC SURGERY CLINICS

www.thoracic.theclinics.com

Consulting Editor
M. BLAIR MARSHALL

February 2018 • Volume 28 • Number 1

ELSEVIER

1600 John F. Kennedy Boulevard • Suite 1800 • Philadelphia, Pennsylvania, 19103-2899

http://www.thoracic.theclinics.com

THORACIC SURGERY CLINICS Volume 28, Number 1
February 2018 ISSN 1547-4127, ISBN-13: 978-0-323-57004-6

Editor: John Vassallo (j.vassallo@elsevier.com)
Developmental Editor: Laura Fisher

Thoracic Surgery Clinics (ISSN 1547-4127) is published quarterly by Elsevier Inc., 360 Park Avenue South, New York, NY 10010-1710. Months of publication are February, May, August, and November. Business and editorial offices: 1600 John F. Kennedy Boulevard, Suite 1800, Philadelphia, PA 19103-2899. Periodicals postage paid at New York, NY, and additional mailing offices. Subscription prices are $373.00 per year (US individuals), $558.00 per year (US institutions), $100.00 per year (US students), $455.00 per year (Canadian individuals), $721.00 per year (Canadian institutions), $225.00 per year (Canadian and international students), $470.00 per year (international individuals), and $721.00 per year (international institutions). Foreign air speed delivery is included in all Clinics' subscription prices. All prices are subject to change without notice. **POSTMASTER:** Send address changes to Thoracic Surgery Clinics, Elsevier Health Sciences Division, Subscription Customer Service, 3251 Riverport Lane, Maryland Heights, MO 63043. **Customer Service (orders, claims, online, change of address): Telephone: 1-800-654-2452 (U.S. and Canada); 314-447-8871 (outside U.S. and Canada). Fax: 314-447-8029. E-mail: journalscustomerservice-usa@elsevier.com (for print support); journalsonlinesupport-usa@elsevier.com (for online support).**

Reprints. For copies of 100 or more, of articles in this publication, please contact Commercial Rights Department, Elsevier Inc., 360 Park Avenue South, New York, NY 10010-1710. Tel: 212-633-3874; Fax: 212-633-3820; E-mail: reprints@elsevier.com.

Thoracic Surgery Clinics is covered in *MEDLINE/PubMed (Index Medicus), EMBASE/Excerpta Medica, Science Citation Index Expanded (SciSearch®), Journal Citation Reports/Science Edition,* and *Current Contents®/Clinical Medicine*.

Contributors

CONSULTING EDITOR

M. BLAIR MARSHALL, MD, FACS
Chief, Division of Thoracic Surgery, Associate Professor, Department of Surgery, Georgetown University Medical Center, Georgetown University School of Medicine, Washington, DC

EDITOR

SHARON BEN-OR, MD
Assistant Professor, Division of Thoracic Surgery, Department of Surgery, Greenville Memorial Hospital, Greenville, South Carolina

AUTHORS

ABBAS E. ABBAS, MD
Professor, Chief, Division of Thoracic Surgery, Department of Thoracic Medicine and Surgery, Temple University Hospital, Fox Chase Cancer Center, Lewis Katz School of Medicine, Philadelphia, Pennsylvania

CARLOS J. ANCIANO, MD
Assistant Professor, Thoracic and Foregut Surgery, Director, Minimally Invasive Thoracic Surgery, Department of Cardiovascular Sciences, East Carolina University, Greenville, North Carolina

MEGUMI ASAI, MD
Chief Resident, General Surgery, Department of Thoracic Surgery, Abington-Jefferson Health, Abington, Pennsylvania

MARVIN D. ATKINS, MD
Resident, Cardiothoracic Surgery, Division of Cardiothoracic Surgery, Hospital of the University of Pennsylvania, Philadelphia, Pennsylvania

CHARLES BAKHOS, MD
Associate Professor, Division of Thoracic Surgery, Department of Thoracic Medicine and Surgery, Temple University Hospital, Fox Chase Cancer Center, Lewis Katz School of Medicine, Philadelphia, Pennsylvania

SHARON BEN-OR, MD
Assistant Professor, Division of Thoracic Surgery, Department of Surgery, Greenville Memorial Hospital, Greenville, South Carolina

MARK F. BERRY, MD
Associate Professor, Department of Cardiothoracic Surgery, Stanford University, Stanford, California

WILLIAM D. BOLTON, MD
Department of Surgery, Division of Thoracic Surgery, University of South Carolina, School of Medicine Greenville, Greenville, South Carolina

TIMOTHY BRAND, MD
Division of Cardiothoracic Surgery, Department of Surgery, The University of North Carolina at Chapel Hill, Chapel Hill, North Carolina

STEPHANIE FULLER, MD, MS
Associate Professor of Surgery, Division of Cardiothoracic Surgery, Perelman School of Medicine University of Pennsylvania, Children's Hospital of Philadelphia, Philadelphia, Pennsylvania

JULIAN GUITRON, MD
Associate Professor of Surgery, Division of Thoracic Surgery, Department of Surgery, University of Cincinnati College of Medicine, Loveland, Ohio

BENJAMIN HAITHCOCK, MD
Division of Cardiothoracic Surgery, Department of Surgery, The University of North Carolina at Chapel Hill, Chapel Hill, North Carolina

DORAID JARRAR, MD
Division of Thoracic Surgery, Perelman School of Medicine University of Pennsylvania, Penn Presbyterian Medical Center, Philadelphia, Pennsylvania

DOUGLAS Z. LIOU, MD
Cardiothoracic Surgery Resident, Department of Cardiothoracic Surgery, Stanford University, Stanford, California

MATTHEW LOW, MD
Department of Surgery, Greenville Health System, Greenville, South Carolina

KATY A. MARINO, MD
Division of Thoracic Surgery, Department of Surgery, The University of Tennessee Health Science Center, Memphis, Tennessee

ANTHONY B. MOZER, MD, MBA
General Surgery Resident, Department of Surgery, East Carolina University, Greenville, North Carolina

AMAR N. MUKERJI, MD
Administrative Chief Resident, Department of Surgery, Bronx-Lebanon Hospital Center, Bronx, New York

ROMAN PETROV, MD
Assistant Professor, Department of Thoracic Medicine and Surgery, Division of Thoracic Surgery, Temple University Hospital, Fox Chase Cancer Center, Lewis Katz School of Medicine, Philadelphia, Pennsylvania

BENJAMIN POWELL, MD
Department of Surgery, Greenville Health System, Greenville, South Carolina

WALTER J. SCOTT, MD, FACS
Professor of Surgery, Sidney Kimmel Medical College, Thomas Jefferson University, Chief, Division of Thoracic Surgery, Abington Jefferson Hospital, Abington, Pennsylvania

GRACE Y. SONG, MD
Division of Thoracic Surgery, Perelman School of Medicine University of Pennsylvania, Penn Presbyterian Medical Center, Philadelphia, Pennsylvania

JAMES E. SPEICHER, MD
Assistant Professor, Thoracic and Foregut Surgery, Department of Cardiovascular Sciences, East Carolina University, Greenville, North Carolina

BENNY WEKSLER, MBA, MD
Eastridge-Cole Professor of Thoracic Oncology, Chief, Division of Thoracic Surgery, Department of Surgery, The University of Tennessee Health Science Center, Memphis, Tennessee

BRIAN WHANG, MD, FACS
Instructor of Surgery, Division of Thoracic Surgery, Brigham and Women's Hospital, Boston, Massachusetts

ANDREA WOLF, MD, MPH
Assistant Professor, Department of Thoracic Surgery, Icahn School of Medicine at Mount Sinai, New York, New York

Contents

Preface: Thoracic Surgery in the Special Care Patient ix

Sharon Ben-Or

Thoracic Surgery in the Pregnant Patient 1

Brian Whang

Thoracic surgeons are sometimes asked to consult on the management of a patient who is pregnant. Conditions commonly encountered are empyema, spontaneous pneumothorax, and diaphragmatic hernia. Lung cancer is rarely seen in pregnancy, but its incidence is rising. Diagnostic imaging and perioperative management involve the navigation of fetal risks and nuances in maternal physiology. Shared decision making within a multidisciplinary framework will optimally guide the course of management.

Thoracic Surgery in Early-Stage Small Cell Lung Cancer 9

Matthew Low and Sharon Ben-Or

Small cell lung cancer (SCLC) has a complex history and remains difficult to treat. Most patients with SCLC present with metastases or extensive stage disease, rendering most not amenable to surgical resection. Until recently, chemoradiotherapy had become the standard of care for all patients with SCLC. However, recent studies have shown improved survival following surgical resection with chemotherapy in patients with early-stage SCLC, specifically those with stage I disease. This article presents the literature on treatment of early-stage SCLC and addresses the question of whether surgery should be considered a viable treatment modality.

Lung Cancer and Lung Transplantation 15

Timothy Brand and Benjamin Haithcock

Lung transplantation remains a viable option for patients with end-stage pulmonary disease. Despite removing the affected organ and replacing both lungs, the risk of lung malignancies still exists. Regardless of the mode of entry, lung cancer affects the prognosis in these patients, and diligence is required.

Lung Resection in the Postpneumonectomy Patient 19

Megumi Asai and Walter J. Scott

Pulmonary resection after pneumonectomy is a reasonable option in selected patients. Wedge resection for single peripheral metachronous disease has the best outcome, with 5-year survival as high as 63%. Current and predicted postoperative cardiopulmonary reserve should be evaluated carefully. Stereotactic body radiotherapy is a promising alternative for inoperable patients.

Thoracic Surgery Considerations in Obese Patients 27

Douglas Z. Liou and Mark F. Berry

The obesity epidemic in the United States has increased greatly over the past several decades, and thoracic surgeons are likely to see obese patients routinely in their practices. Obesity has direct deleterious health effects such as metabolic disorder and cardiovascular disease and is associated with many cancers. Obese patients who need thoracic surgery pose practical challenges to many of the routine elements in perioperative management. Preoperative assessment of obesity-related comorbid conditions and risk stratification for surgery, thorough intraoperative planning for anesthesia and surgery, and postoperative strategies to optimize pulmonary hygiene and mobility minimize the risk of adverse outcomes.

Thoracic Surgery Considerations in the Child and Young Adult **43**

Marvin D. Atkins and Stephanie Fuller

Vascular rings and slings may represent life-threatening compression of the esophagus and trachea. Such anatomic variants, although rare, are encountered by all thoracic surgeons in the scope of their practice at some time. The thoracic surgeon, whether treating such patients in the practice of congenital heart surgery or in the practice of adult cardiac or thoracic surgery, must have a requisite understanding of such anatomic variants, their diagnostic workup and radiologic interpretation, as well as their surgical management. Primary tracheobronchial disorders are also frequently encountered in the scope of a thoracic surgical practice and also are discussed.

Esophagectomy After Weight-Reduction Surgery **53**

Katy A. Marino and Benny Weksler

Obesity is now epidemic worldwide, and an increasing number of patients have undergone a weight-loss procedure. Although obesity is a risk factor for esophageal cancer, there are few reports on esophagectomy after bariatric procedures. Careful understanding of the patient's gastroesophageal anatomy as a result of the bariatric procedure and attention to the creation of the esophageal replacement conduit are fundamental for the success of esophagectomy after bariatric surgery.

Thoracic Surgery Considerations in the Mentally Ill or Handicapped Patient **59**

Anthony B. Mozer, James E. Speicher, and Carlos J. Anciano

 Video content accompanies this article at http://www.thoracic.theclinics.com.

Increasing prevalence of mentally ill and handicapped populations requiring surgical thoracic interventions has brought to light their worse associated morbidity and mortality. Baseline functional status, caretaker environment, and mental limitations in day-to-day life have an impact in the short and long term from these interventions. Aggressive perioperative care, multispecialty approach, technical aspects, palliative procedures, and ethical considerations all play a part in improving outcomes. In this article real cases are presented illustrating points of care and situations for discussion.

Management of Lung Cancer with Concomitant Cardiac Disease **69**

Benjamin Powell and William D. Bolton

This article discusses the numerous issues surrounding lung cancer treatment in patients with concomitant cardiac disease. It also addresses the preoperative workup of these patients and the specifics of surgical intervention.

Management of Malignant Lung Entrapment, the Oncothorax 81

Roman Petrov, Charles Bakhos, and Abbas E. Abbas

Pleural metastasis is a common occurrence in up to 30% of patients with metastatic cancer. When lung entrapment and loculation of fluid occur, treatment is more difficult and we have named this condition "oncothorax." The malignant adhesions that entrap the lung in an oncothorax are not typically amenable to surgical decortication. The standard approach for managing these patients is to place an indwelling catheter. Other options may include pleurectomy and decortication, intrapleural hyperthermic chemoperfusion, and intrapleural photodynamic therapy. However, these procedures should be provided selectively depending on patient performance status, extent of metastatic disease, and level of experience.

Empyema from Obstructing Lung Cancer 91

Julian Guitron

Pleural collections on the side of an obstructing bronchial cancer pose a particular challenge. All efforts should be placed into determining whether the collection is malignant or paramalignant with its significant implications on cancer staging. This article discusses various diagnostic modalities and therapeutic interventions needed for the optimal management of patients presenting with this situation. The order of interventions is dictated by the individual circumstances that patients present with, often requiring the pleural interventions to take place ahead of the bronchial obstruction management.

Synchronous Esophageal and Lung Cancer 97

Amar N. Mukerji and Andrea Wolf

Synchronous lung and esophageal cancers are rare but represent a unique challenge to thoracic surgeons. The literature is limited but series describe long-term survival with curative surgery for concomitant esophageal and lung cancer. Preoperative risk assessment is critical because surgical resection of both cancers requires adequate cardiopulmonary function and performance status. Chemotherapy and radiation are used as adjuvant therapy or as primary treatment of unresectable lesions. Although long-term survival for patients with concomitant lung and esophageal cancer is lower than that of patients with either one alone, survival with curative surgery is higher than that of patients with metastatic disease of either primary.

Thoracic Surgery in Patients with AIDS 105

Doraid Jarrar and Grace Y. Song

The picture of human immunodeficiency virus (HIV)–infected patients has changed dramatically since the original description in 1981. The introduction of antiretroviral drugs in 1987 and combination antiretroviral therapy has decreased mortality by as much as 80%. We now see patients in their 60s and 70s, having lived decades with HIV and living a normal live. As outlined in the article, despite good viral control, patients with HIV may present with solid organ cancers earlier than noninfected patients and are also prone to other complications of their disease that may require the attention of a thoracic surgeon.

THORACIC SURGERY CLINICS

FORTHCOMING ISSUES

May 2018
Fundamentals of Airway Surgery, Part I
Jean Deslauriers, Farid M. Shamji, and Bill Nelems, *Editors*

August 2018
Fundamentals of Airway Surgery, Part II
Jean Deslauriers, Farid M. Shamji, and Bill Nelems, *Editors*

November 2018
Novel Options in the Management of Foregut Disease
Brian Louie, *Editor*

RECENT ISSUES

November 2017
Single-port/Uniportal Video-Assisted Thoracic Surgery
Gaetano Rocco, *Editor*

August 2017
Quality in Thoracic Surgery
Felix G. Fernandez, *Editor*

May 2017
Disorders of the Chest Wall
Henning A. Gaissert, *Editor*

RELATED INTEREST

Surgical Clinics, December 2017 (Vol. 97, Issue 6)
Surgical Critical Care
Cynthia L. Talley, *Editor*
Available at: http://www.surgical.theclinics.com

Preface

Thoracic Surgery in the Special Care Patient

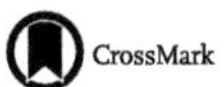

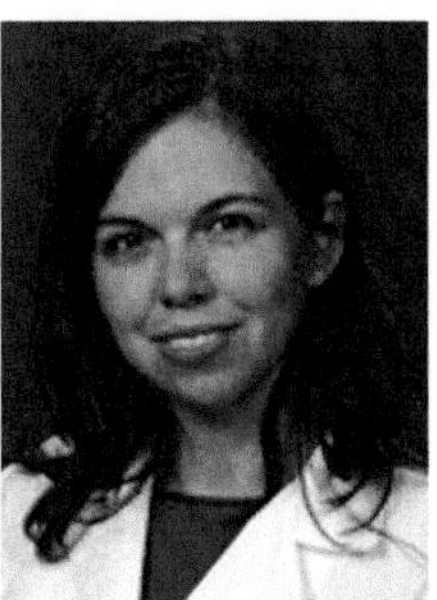

Sharon Ben-Or, MD
Editor

Every thoracic surgeon has encountered a patient whose problem is outside of the box, a clinical conundrum. Often, the diagnosis and workup can be as vexing as formulating a treatment plan. These patients require thoughtful and methodical care often with the input of multiple physicians from multiple subspecialties. Evidence for these disease processes exists, but guidelines are scarce. From the pregnant patient to the lung transplant recipient with lung cancer to the patient who underwent weight reduction surgery with esophageal cancer, these unique patients require the attention and innovation of a thoracic surgeon who sometimes has to push the envelope in order to treat the patient.

This issue of *Thoracic Surgery Clinics* focuses on the complex diagnoses of these special care patients that do not fit any particular category. These cases are rarely encountered but are always memorable. I would like to thank each contributor for taking the time to reflect on their own past experiences and pitfalls of each of these patients. As we pull back the curtain on these rare clinical challenges, we hope to shed light on how to appropriately treat these unforgettable patients.

Sharon Ben-Or, MD
Division of Thoracic Surgery
Department of Surgery
Greenville Memorial Hospital
890 West Faris Road, Suite 320
Greenville, SC 29605, USA

E-mail address:
SBen-Or@ghs.org

Thorac Surg Clin 28 (2018) ix
http://dx.doi.org/10.1016/j.thorsurg.2017.09.006
1547-4127/18/

Thoracic Surgery in the Pregnant Patient

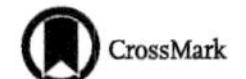

Brian Whang, MD

KEYWORDS

- Pregnancy • Thoracic surgery • Gestational cancer • Empyema • Pneumothorax
- Diaphragmatic hernia

KEY POINTS

- Ionizing radiation affects the fetus depending on dose and timing of exposure. The use of radiographs, CT, and ultrasound is acceptable during pregnancy. MRI may be used in a limited fashion. PET should not be used until after delivery.
- Surgery using general anesthesia can be safely performed after the first trimester. There are cardiovascular, pulmonary, and gastrointestinal changes in pregnancy that must be considered in the conduct of surgery. Ideal pain management makes use of epidural anesthesia while limiting reliance on opiate medications.
- Empyema is a frequent complication of pneumonia during pregnancy, and video-assisted thoracoscopic surgery drainage can be safely performed. Spontaneous pneumothorax has a high rate of recurrence during pregnancy. Diaphragmatic hernia may be exacerbated while gestation progresses, which can lead to incarceration and strangulation.
- Lung cancer is rare during pregnancy, but the incidence is rising. Lung cancer reaches an advanced stage when recognized. Occasions for curative surgery are infrequent, and chemotherapy is the mainstay of treatment. There is a limited role for radiotherapy.
- Shared decision making should be a goal throughout the management of the pregnant thoracic patient.

INTRODUCTION

Although an uncommon occurrence, the thoracic surgeon may sometimes be asked to consult on the management of a patient who is pregnant. There are no specific diseases that are uniquely germane to pregnancy in the thoracic wheelhouse, although several common conditions are known to afflict pregnant women with notable frequency, such as empyema, spontaneous pneumothorax, and diaphragmatic hernia.[1–13] Neoplasms of the chest may also be encountered. Increased smoking among women and delayed childbearing are expected to contribute to a rise in gestational cancer, including that of lung cancer.[14–18] Given the concerns for both mother and fetus, many aspects of management, from diagnosis to treatment, are influenced by the relative merits and risks for both entities. This overview illustrates such considerations when approaching diagnostic imaging, perioperative care, and predominant thoracic conditions described in the literature, with particular attention paid to the treatment of cancer. The unifying principle of all these endeavors should be shared decision-making, in which the patient is sufficiently informed and supported to make choices that are congruous with her values and beliefs.[15,17,19–21]

DIAGNOSTIC IMAGING

The use of radiographs and CT is pervasive in the standard work-up of thoracic patients. The deleterious effects of ionizing radiation on the fetus,

Disclosure Statement: There are no disclosures or conflicts of interest.

Division of Thoracic Surgery, Brigham and Women's Hospital, 75 Francis Street, Boston, MA 02115, USA
E-mail address: bwhang@bwh.harvard.edu

Thorac Surg Clin 28 (2018) 1–7
https://doi.org/10.1016/j.thorsurg.2017.08.002
1547-4127/18/

however, are well documented, based on studies of atomic bomb survivors, patients exposed to medical radiation, and animal models.[22] During the first 2 weeks after conception, the irradiated embryo either dies or undergoes normal development, following the all-or-nothing rule.[14,15] The 3-week to 8-week period of early organogenesis that follows is keenly sensitive to the effects of radiation. Death, developmental malformations, and growth retardation may occur with doses as low as 50 mGy to 250 mGy. Fetal doses of 100 mGy to 250 mGy are generally cited as thresholds for such teratogenicity.[15,22,23] During weeks 8 to 15, there is a high risk of severe mental retardation at doses of 60 mGy to 310 mGy as well as microcephaly over a threshold of 200 mGy. At 16 weeks to 25 weeks, a low risk for severe mental retardation exists at doses over 250 mGy.[23] After 25 weeks, the deterministic effects are thought to be insignificant.[17] The stochastic effects include a 6.4% risk of carcinogenesis from childhood to young adulthood per gray of gestational radiation exposure.[24]

Fortunately, diagnostic radiography can be safely used when abiding by limitations on dose, gestational age, and radiation field.[14,15,17,25–27] When using the principle of as-low-as-reasonably-achievable (ALARA), a routine chest CT delivers indirect fetal exposure that is less than 0.2 mGy.[15,28] The dose of a chest radiograph is estimated at 0.0004 mGy.[15] Given these small doses, external shielding is not necessary, although the patient may find it reassuring.[22] Internal shielding is also achievable through the ingestion of oral barium.[29] In addition, the use of iodinated intravenous (IV) contrast has not been shown to be teratogenic. Because it can cross the placenta, however, there is the theoretic risk of neonatal hypothyroidism. Again, this is not supported by the literature. Nonetheless, its use should be restricted to when absolutely necessary.[23]

MRI seems to be an attractive option, given its clinical utility and independence from ionizing radiation. Some investigators advocate its use as a safe and appropriate modality for metastatic work-up.[20,25] No studies have yet to demonstrate harm to the fetus. There are concerns, however, over the potential for tissue heating and other biological insults as well as auditory damage produced by varying gradient electromagnetic fields.[22] Consequently, current guidelines recommend the use of MRI only when there are no suitable alternatives, the information is likely to affect patient care, and the study cannot wait until after the completion of pregnancy.[27,30] Similarly, although there are no documented teratogenic effects of gadolinium in humans, its use is also restricted by the same criteria, and there must be collaboration between the radiologist and referring physician.[30]

PET is another imaging modality commonly used in the work-up of thoracic malignancy, but it cannot be recommended during pregnancy. This is due to the prohibitive amount of radiation exposure from the passage of fludeoxyglucose F 18 across the placenta.[31] Even after delivery, breastfeeding must be temporarily suspended due to the high concentration of Fludeoxyglucose F 18 in breast milk.[32]

Ultrasound has the best safety profile of all, and it has particular clinical utility in image-guided procedures, such as thoracentesis and percutaneous biopsy of cervical and supraclavicular lymph nodes. Loculated pleural and pericardial effusions can be precisely investigated, and chest wall masses can often be examined with sufficient clarity. Ultrasound can also be a useful adjunct in the evaluation of abdominopelvic disease.[25,27]

PERIOPERATIVE ISSUES

Nonobstetric surgery is performed on 0.5% to 2% of pregnant women in North America per year.[33] Anesthetic agents are potentially teratogenic, so the use of general anesthesia is best avoided until the second trimester.[34] The actual risk of spontaneous abortion is 1% to 10% in the first trimester,[17,35] but this risk becomes comparable to the normal miscarriage rate when appendectomies are excluded. Relative risk for low birth weight and premature labor is only slightly increased throughout gestation (1.5–2.0),[36] although it is relatively higher during the third trimester.[3] As with miscarriage, the rate of premature labor is also affected by surgical site; it is more common with lower abdominal or pelvic surgeries.[37] The safety and feasibility of thoracic surgical intervention have been well documented in the literature, including that of video-assisted thoracoscopic surgery (VATS).[2,3,10,27,38–41] The use of CO_2 insufflation in VATS, however, has not yet been reported. If surgery cannot be delayed until the onset of fetal maturity, then the risk profile favors proceeding in the interest of maternal health.[17]

The fetal and maternal safety at hand is the salutary effect of modern anesthetic and operative management that has been mindful of several nuances in pregnant physiology. In the mother, there is increased blood volume, heart rate, and cardiac output. This is accompanied by supine hypotension, elevated diaphragm, decreased pulmonary functional residual capacity, delayed gastric emptying, and hypervascularity of the respiratory tract mucosa.[37] Aspiration of gastric contents is a particular risk, and rapid sequence or awake intubation is sometimes used. H_2-blockers are recommended to decrease gastric secretions and acidity.[34] Preeclampsia is also known to potentiate airway edema and small airway closure.[38,39]

The high maternal metabolic rate and increased oxygen consumption are necessary for adequate placental blood supply. Therefore, arterial blood gases are closely monitored, and inhaled fraction of inspired oxygen must be adjusted accordingly, especially when single-lung ventilation is used. Coughing and straining are also avoided on induction and extubation to limit downstream insults to fetal oxygenation.[3,38,39] Aortocaval compression from the gravid uterus is another potential threat to the placental blood supply.[3,30] Although a slight left lateral decubitus maneuver is often used when a patient is supine, thoracic procedures requiring a left-sided approach require that the right side be placed down. Fortunately, a full lateral decubitus position still allows for decompression of retroperitoneal structures. Hypotension must be aggressively treated using IV fluids, phenylephrine, or ephedrine.[34] Continuous fetal monitoring is maintained throughout the procedure, and arrangements for caesarean delivery can be made as a precaution.[39]

Epidural anesthesia can be implemented for postoperative pain control to limit the use of opioid medications, which can contribute to maternal respiratory depression. There is also a concern for fetal tolerance and addiction with prolonged opioid use.[15] Acetaminophen is another safe alternative that can be administered throughout pregnancy. On the other hand, nonsteroidal anti-inflammatory drugs, although nonteratogenic, are nonetheless associated with premature closure of the ductus arteriosus, oligohydramnios, and prolonged labor; their use should be limited and accompanied by close observation.[17]

PREDOMINANT THORACIC CONDITIONS SEEN DURING PREGNANCY

Empyema

Although the prevalence of pneumonia in pregnant patients is similar to that of nonpregnant controls, the risk of maternal complications is increased. Examples include respiratory failure (10%–20%), bacteremia (16%), and empyema (8%).[2,42,43] Aside from the dire maternal consequences, adverse fetal effects include preterm labor and birth, low birth weight, and neonatal mortality.[42] By assuming a definitive role in the management of empyema, the thoracic surgeon is therefore poised to avert further deterioration in this subset of patients. VATS drainage and decortication have been documented as a safe and effective remedy in pregnant patients that can promptly curtail these patients' overall hospital course.[2,43,44] The feasibility of awake VATS decortication has also been demonstrated in the nonpregnant population, which may eventually validate its applicability during the first trimester.[45] Otherwise, the use of fibrinolytic agents via tube thoracostomy has also shown satisfactory results that are without adverse maternal or fetal effects. Although the data are limited to case reports, the increases in drainage after 2 to 3 administrations of intrapleural streptokinase were instrumental in bringing about the complete resolution of these cases of empyema.[1,46]

Spontaneous Pneumothorax

Primary spontaneous pneumothorax is known to have a recurrence rate of approximately 30% after the first episode. Pregnant patients are even more disposed to recur, with a rate of 44%.[8] Moreover, it is likely to happen again during pregnancy or at the time of delivery.[8,47] One such patient presented with 7 pneumothoraces over 2 separate pregnancies. In the end, she underwent thoracoscopic interventions on each side, followed by tubal ligation.[4] Just as in the nonpregnant population, surgical observation and CT scanning have demonstrated the presence of apical blebs. These are thought to rupture as a result of changes in maternal respiratory physiology: rising tidal volumes, increased respiratory rate, and a 70% increase in alveolar ventilation.[8]

VATS with bleb resection and pleurodesis have been performed safely and effectively; no intrapartum recurrences have been reported thus far.[8] Current guidelines now suggest, however, postponing this surgery until after delivery.[7]

Even the insertion of chest tubes has been supplanted in favor of observation for asymptomatic, small (<2 cm) pneumothoraces, and simple aspiration for larger ones. A success rate of 80% has been quoted for the latter.[8] Tube thoracostomy is reserved for patients who demonstrate recurrence after aspiration.[7,8] Moreover, elective assisted delivery with an epidural or caesarean section under regional anesthesia is recommended to avoid the punctuated surges in intrathoracic pressure associated with spontaneous childbirth. The stakes involved at parturition, and the limited capacity for a reliable examination in cases of pneumothorax, make the deliberate path of elective delivery a safer option.[7,8]

Two types of secondary spontaneous pneumothorax in pregnancy have also been documented in the literature. Warren and colleagues[5] describe a 32-year-old woman who presented with bilateral pneumothoraces during her 12th week of gestation. Sequential thoracotomies ultimately diagnosed lymphangiomyomatosis. Hormonal therapy was deferred until after completion of pregnancy. The second group of secondary spontaneous pneumothorax consists of 5 cases of ectopic deciduosis. Like its counterpart, catamenial pneumothorax, this is due to endometriosis-derived pulmonary implantation, and recurrence is high. Ectopic deciduosis, however, is not tied to menstruation, and it manages to flourish despite the state of amenorrhea created by pregnancy.[9,10] Pneumothorax is thought to be related to the structural weakening of lung tissue caused by the decidualization of endometriosis.[9] Treatment involves surgical extirpation of involved lung, pleurodesis, pleurectomy, closure of diaphragmatic fenestrations, and hormonal therapy.[9,10]

Diaphragmatic Hernia

Among pregnant women, 50% to 80% complain of heartburn, and there seems to be a cumulative effect of multiple pregnancies on the exacerbation of reflux.[48] The increase in intra-abdominal pressure imposed by the growing uterus weakens diaphragmatic attachments to the esophagus until an acquired hiatal hernia is formed.[11] High progesterone levels are also thought to contribute to the laxity of the diaphragm and associated ligaments.[12]

When clinically advanced, the most common presenting symptoms are nausea and vomiting, abdominal pain, and dyspnea. Understandably, these are nonspecific and are often confused with the constellation of pregnancy-related maladies. Consequently, 50% of cases are misdiagnosed and are prevented from further work-up, which should include imaging.[12] Nausea itself, however, is usually limited to the first 12 weeks of normal pregnancy, except in cases of hyperemesis gravidarum. By contrast, most patients with symptomatic diaphragmatic hernia present with nausea in the third trimester.[12]

Once detected, symptomatic defects are ideally repaired during the second trimester. After this window, especially at the time of delivery, diaphragmatic rents are further exacerbated by the enlarging uterus and vigorous contractions of labor. Moreover, the intrathoracic excursion of abdominal viscera becomes less reducible and more prone to strangulation.[12,13] Conservative management is usually sufficient for uncomplicated hernias discovered only by the third trimester. Surgical repair can then immediately follow delivery by caesarean section. Cases of obstruction or volvulus, however, should be urgently repaired, regardless of gestational age, given the fetal and maternal mortality rate of 35% to 50%.[12]

LUNG CANCER IN PREGNANCY

The overall incidence of cancer is estimated at 1 in 1000 to 1500 pregnancies.[14,15,18,26] The most common types of malignancies are breast cancer, cervical cancer, melanoma, thyroid cancer, and Hodgkins lymphoma.[14–17] When matched by age, the incidence of malignancies is the same among pregnant and nonpregnant women.[14,49] Pregnancy itself is not known to be a risk factor for malignancy.[15] By comparison, lung cancer is exceedingly rare, and there are only 60 cases documented in the literature.[27] Nonetheless, a majority come from the past 20 years,[20,38] which raises the possibility that the incidence is climbing. Two reasons have been suggested for this finding. One is the proliferation of cigarette smokers among young women.[14,38,50] The other is the rise in maternal age as childbearing is increasingly being experienced beyond the third decade of life.[14–18] The median age at diagnosis of lung cancer has been reported between 36 years and 39 years, with a median gestational age of 27 to 29 weeks. Non–small cell lung cancer comprises the majority of cases, with adenocarcinoma the most frequent type.[25,27]

Advanced disease is the norm at diagnosis, with 80% to 90% of cases presenting at stage III or stage IV.[20,25] Although this may be similar to the discovery of lung cancer in the nonpregnant population, the challenge is compounded by the nonspecific nature of some of the signs and symptoms, such as fatigue, anemia, and nausea, within the clinical context of pregnancy.[14] More distinct findings like cough, hemoptysis, and bone pain are cited as the most common on reaching presentation.[15] Low level of suspicion and apprehension in proceeding with radiological tests and procedures are additional impediments to diagnosis.[27] Median survival is 4 months, although stage for stage, maternal outcome does not differ from that of nonpregnant patients.[15,17,27] Thus far, no data indicate that lung cancer behaves in a fundamentally unique way during pregnancy.[27] Furthermore, termination of pregnancy has not been shown to improve survival.[14,15,25,26]

Attempts at curative surgery are infrequent, given the advanced stage at which gestational lung cancer is usually diagnosed, but this should still be pursued using the standard clinical indications.[15] Most patients undergoing resection have done so during the postpartum period, but there is 1 documented case of a video-assisted thoracoscopic lobectomy successfully performed during the second trimester of pregnancy.[20,27,40,51] By and large, surgery during pregnancy has been limited to minor palliative endeavors and diagnostic procedures, such as bronchoscopy.

Chemotherapy is the cornerstone of gestational lung cancer treatment, as it is for most malignancies discovered during pregnancy.[14–21,25–27,37,51–53] Although all agents can cross the placenta, adverse effects are mainly confined to their use during the first trimester.[27] Fetal malformation due to chemotherapy ranges between 12.7% and 17%, whereas low birth weight is approximately 40%.[53] The risks of miscarriage and fetal malformation can be reduced from 20% to 1% when restricting chemotherapy to the second and third trimesters, so it is preferable to postpone this treatment beyond the first trimester whenever possible.[15,17] Both cisplatin and carboplatin have been administered with similar efficacy, although cisplatin has a worse fetal toxicity profile.[14,20,27] Taxanes also seem to demonstrate acceptable safety during the second and third trimesters.[54] Platinum-based regimens used in combination with taxanes have been used with relative safety, although with tepid results.[20,27] Disappointing responses may be due to differences in maternal pharmacokinetics. For example, plasma binding proteins are raised during pregnancy, which may decrease the active fraction of agents, such as taxanes and vinorelbine, which are tightly bound to plasma proteins. Consequently, standard dosing regimens may be underestimated, although no survival differences have been appreciated in comparison to stage-matched cohorts.[27] Regardless of agent used, delivery should be delayed for 2 weeks to 3 weeks after the completion of chemotherapy so that there is sufficient time for maternal bone marrow recovery and for fetal drug excretion.[17]

The recent success of tyrosine kinase inhibitors in the targeted treatment of lung cancer has introduced enthusiasm for their expanded use. There is limited evidence, however, regarding their application during pregnancy, due to teratogenic concerns with imatinib mesylate.[17] Nonetheless, 5 cases documenting the use of erlotinib, gefitinib, and crizotinib have demonstrated no adverse fetal effects, albeit with no significant clinical response.[25,27,55] Although preclinical models for erlotinib have failed to show an association with miscarriage or teratogenicity, there is not yet enough evidence to condone its use during pregnancy.[20]

The use of radiotherapy is more problematic than in diagnostic imaging because of the much higher doses that are typically used. Its curative application is generally seen as a contraindication during gestation, and it is usually deferred until the postpartum period.[15,27,56] Its role in palliation is more accepted, however, for distant sites, such as the brain, neck, and distal bones.[20,27,56] The possibility that stereotactic body radiation therapy might offer a safe alternative for intrathoracic disease has not yet been described, although there is some precedent in the use of stereotactic radiosurgery for lesions of the brain.[57–60] Fetal dose exposure should not exceed 100 mGy to 200 mGy, and the radiation oncologist ideally shares planning with an experienced medical physicist.[14,15] Calculation of fetal dose requires attention to several factors: size of the radiation field, target dose, the unique properties of the radiation device, fetal size and position, and projected growth of the fetus over the duration of treatment.[14] Shielding, modification of technique, and the use of low fractional doses over a longer time period are important adjuncts to reducing fetal exposure.[14]

In the limited number of reported cases of gestational lung cancer, 26% have demonstrated vertical transmission to the placenta, whereas the incidence of fetal metastasis approaches 7%.[20,27] Small cell lung cancer is implicated in a majority of both sites. These fetal metastases have involved the scalp, brain, liver, and lung. Encouragingly, none of the patients treated with chemotherapy yielded placental or fetal metastases. It has been recommended that after delivery, the placenta and umbilical cord should be submitted for histopathology and cytology, respectively, and that neonates should be examined for cutaneous lesions and organomegaly. Absent these findings, close observation is still warranted thereafter.[61]

SHARED DECISION MAKING

The dynamics involved in the management of thoracic disease within the context of pregnancy are entrenched in risk-benefit decisions at every turn. Rote patient adherence should be avoided when vague probabilities and competing variables are the currency for emotionally invested consequences. Optimal care requires conscious and deliberate agency of the patient in forming these decisions, because the acceptability of their outcomes may be intrinsically tied to their values and beliefs. In the unfortunate circumstance of lung cancer, termination of pregnancy is often part of a legitimate set of considerations that defy the application of treatment algorithms. Pregnant patients are ideally served when they can make thoroughly informed choices based on best medical knowledge and psychosocial support. In these situations, the thoracic surgeon may not be enough. A multidisciplinary team that consists of allied medical personnel, therapists, and spiritual advisors can offer smoother passage of an otherwise vexing ordeal.[14,15,17,20]

REFERENCES

1. Ulutas H, Yekeler E, Ali Sak ZH, et al. Fibrinolytic therapy for parapneumonic empyema during pregnancy. Respir Med Case Rep 2012;5:55–8.
2. Oshodi T, Carlan SJ, Busowski M, et al. Video assisted thoracic surgery in a second trimester pregnant woman with thoracic empyema: a case report. J Reprod Med 2015;60(3–4):172–4.
3. Mitsunari H, Yamagata K, Sakuma S. Anesthetic management of thoracotomy for spontaneous pneumothorax in a pregnant woman. Int J Obstet Anesth 2008;17(1):85–6.
4. Sills ES, Meinecke HM, Dixson GR, et al. Management approach for recurrent spontaneous pneumothorax in consecutive pregnancies based on clinical and radiographic findings. J Cardiothorac Surg 2006;1:35.
5. Warren SE, Lee D, Martin V, et al. Pulmonary lymphangiomyomatosis causing bilateral pneumothorax during pregnancy. Ann Thorac Surg 1993; 55:998–1000.
6. Nwaejike N, Elbur E, Rammohan KS, et al. Should pregnant patients with a recurrent or persistent pneumothorax undergo surgery? Interact Cardiovasc Thorac Surg 2013;17(6):988–90.
7. MacDuff A, Arnold A, Harvey J. Management of spontaneous pneumothorax: british thoracic society pleural disease Guideline 2010. Thorax 2010; 65(Suppl 2):ii18–31.
8. Lal A, Anderson G, Cowen M, et al. Pneumothorax and pregnancy. Chest 2007;132(3):1044e8.
9. Dudek W, Schreiner W, Strehl J, et al. Spontaneous pneumothorax due to ectopic deciduosis: a case report. Thorac Cardiovasc Surg Rep 2014;3(1):58–60.
10. Kim YD, Min KO, Moon SW. Thoracoscopic treatment of recurrent pneumothorax in a pregnant woman: a case of ectopic deciduosis. Thorac Cardiovasc Surg 2010;58(7):429–30.
11. Baue AE, Naunheim KS. Hiatal hernia and gastroesophageal reflux. In: Baue AE, Geha AS, Hammond GL, et al, editors. Glenn's thoracic and cardiovascular surgery. 5th edition. East Norwalk (CT): Appleton & Lange; 1991. p. 683.
12. Chen Y, Hou Q, Zhang Z, et al. Diaphragmatic hernia during pregnancy: a case report with a review of the literature from the past 50 years. J Obstet Gynaecol Res 2011;37(7):709–14.
13. Kurzel RB, Naunheim KS, Schwartz RA. Repair of symptomatic diaphragmatic hernia during pregnancy. Am J Obstet Gynecol 1988;71(6 Pt 1):869–71.
14. Voulgaris E, Pentheroudakis G, Pavlidis N. Cancer and pregnancy: a comprehensive review. Surg Oncol 2011;20(4):e175–85.
15. Pentheroudakis G, Pavlidis N. Cancer and pregnancy: poena magna, not anymore. Eur J Cancer 2006;42(2):126–40.
16. Antonelli NM, Dotters DJ, Katz VL, et al. Cancer in pregnancy: a review of the literature. Part I–II. Obstet Gynecol Surv 1996;51:125–42.
17. Pereg D, Koren G, Lishner M. Cancer in pregnancy: gaps, challenges and solutions. Cancer Treat Rev 2008;34(4):302–12.
18. Koren G, Lishner M, Santiago S, editors. The Motherisk guide to cancer in pregnancy and lactation. 2nd edition. Toronto: Motherisk Program; 2005.
19. Eisinger F, Noizet A. Breast cancer and pregnancy: decision making and the point of view of the mother. Bull Cancer 2002;89:755–67.
20. Azim HA, Peccatori FA, Pavlidis N. Lung cancer in the pregnant woman: to treat or not to treat, that is the question. Lung Cancer 2010;67(3):251–6.
21. Chervenak FA, McCullough LB, Knapp RC, et al. A clinically comprehensive ethical framework for offering and recommending cancer treatment before and during pregnancy. Cancer 2004;100:215–22.
22. Litmanovich DE, Tack D, Lee KS, et al. Cardiothoracic imaging in the pregnant patient. J Thorac Imaging 2014;29(1):38–49.
23. American College of Radiology. ACR-SPR Practice guideline for imaging pregnant and potentially pregnant adolescents or women with ionizing radiation. Reston (VA): ACR Committee on Drugs and Contrast Media; 2013.
24. Mole RH. Childhood cancer after prenatal exosure to diagnostic X-ray examinations in Britain. Br J Cancer 1990;62:152–68.
25. Sarıman N, Levent E, Yener NA, et al. Lung cancer and pregnancy. Lung Cancer 2013;79(3):321–3.
26. Pavlidis NA. Coexistence of pregnancy and malignancy. Oncologist 2002;7:279–87.
27. Boussios S, Han SN, Fruscio R, et al. Lung cancer in pregnancy: report of nine cases from an international collaborative study. Lung Cancer 2013;82(3): 499–505.
28. Litmanovich D, Tack D, Lin PJ, et al. Female breast, lung, and pelvic organ radiation from dose-reduced 64-MDCT thoracic examination protocols: a phantom study. Am J Roentgenol 2011;197:929–34.
29. Yousefzadeh DK, Ward MB, Reft C. Internal barium shielding to minimize fetal irradiation in spiral chest CT: a phantom simulation experiment. Radiology 2006;239:751–8.

30. Kanal E, Barkovich AJ, Bell C, et al. ACR guidance document for safe MR practices: 2007. Am J Roentgenol 2007;188:1447–74.
31. Benveniste H, Fowler JS, Rooney WD, et al. Maternal–fetal in vivo imaging: a combined PET and MRI study. J Nucl Med 2003;44:1522–30.
32. Hicks RJ, Binns D, Stabin MG. Pattern of uptake and excretion of (18)F-FDG in the lactating breast. J Nucl Med 2001;42:1238–42.
33. Leicht CH. Anesthesia for the pregnant patient undergoing non-obstetric surgery. Anesth Clin North Am 1990;8:131–41.
34. Van de Velde M, De Buck F. Anesthesia for non-obstetric surgery in the pregnant patient. Minerva Anestesiol 2007;73:235–40.
35. Duncan P, Pope W, Cohen M, et al. Foetal risk of anesthesia and surgery during pregnancy. Anesthesiology 1986;64:790–4.
36. Mazze R, Kallen B. Reproductive outcome after anesthesia and operation during pregnancy: a registry study of 5405 cases. Am J Obstet Gynecol 1989;161:1178–85.
37. Petrek JA. Breast cancer during pregnancy. Cancer 1994;74:518–27.
38. Burlacu CL, Fitzpatrick C, Carey M. Anaesthesia for caesarean section in a woman with lung cancer: case report and review. Int J Obstet Anesth 2007; 16:50–62.
39. Webster JA, Self DD. Anesthesia for pericardial window in a pregnant patient with cardiac tamponade and mediastinal mass. Can J Anaesth 2003;50(8): 815–8.
40. Kim JW, Kim JS, Cho JY, et al. Successful video-assisted thoracoscopic lobectomy in a pregnant woman with lung cancer. Lung Cancer 2014;85(2): 331–4.
41. Şahin M, Kocaman G, Özkan M. Resection of esophageal carcinoma during pregnancy. Ann Thorac Surg 2015;99(1):333–5.
42. Goodnight WH, Soper DE. Pneumonia in pregnancy. Crit Care Med 2005;33(10 Suppl):S390–7.
43. Madinger NE, Creenspoon J, Ellrodt AG. Pneumonia during pregnancy: has modern technology improved maternal and fetal outcome? Am J Obstet Gynecol 1989;161:657–62.
44. Gossot D, Stern JB, Galetta D, et al. Thoracoscopic management of postpneumonectomy empyema. Ann Thorac Surg 2004;78:273–6.
45. Tacconi F, Pompeo E, Pabbi E, et al. Awake video-assisted pleural decortication for empyema thoracis. Eur J Cardiothorac Surg 2010;37:594–601.
46. Nir S, Gadi L, Mony S, et al. Successful use of streptokinase for the treatment of empyema thoracis during advanced pregnancy: a case report. Respir Med 2009;2:21e4.
47. Terndrup TE, Bosco SF, McLean ER. Spontaneous pneumothorax complicating pregnancy: case report and review of the literature. J Emerg Med 1989;7: 245e8.
48. Bainbridge ET, Temple JG, Nicholas SP, et al. Symptomatic gastro-oesophageal reflux in pregnancy: a comparative study of white Europeans and Asians in Birmingham. Br J Clin Pract 1983;37(2):53–7.
49. Liberman L, Giess CS, Dershaw DD, et al. Imaging of pregnancy-associated breast cancer. Radiology 1994;191(1):245e8.
50. Lader D, Goddard E. Smoking-related behaviour and attitudes 2003. London: Office for National Statistics; 2004. Crown Copyright.
51. Garrido M, Clavero J, Huete A, et al. Prolonged survival of a woman with lung cancer diagnosed and treated with chemotherapy during pregnancy. Review of cases reported. Lung Cancer 2008;60: 285–90.
52. Janne PA, Rodriguez-Thompson D, Metcalf DR, et al. Chemotherapy for a patient with advanced non-small cell lung cancer during pregnancy: a case report and a review of chemotherapy treatment during pregnancy. Oncology 2001;61:175–83.
53. Abdel-Hady el-S, Hemida RA, Gamal A, et al. Cancer during pregnancy: perinatal outcome after in utero exposure to chemotherapy. Arch Gynecol Obstet 2012;286:283–6.
54. Mir O, Berveiller P, Goffinet F, et al. Taxanes for breast cancer during pregnancy: a systematic review. Ann Oncol 2010;21:425–6.
55. Zambelli A, Prada GA, Fregoni V, et al. Erlotinib administration for advanced non-small cell lung cancer during the first 2 months of unrecognized pregnancy. Lung Cancer 2008;60(3):455–7.
56. Orecchia R, Lucignani G, Tosi G. Prenatal irradiation and pregnancy: the effects of diagnostic imaging and radiation therapy. Recent Results Cancer Res 2008;178:3–20.
57. Ioffe V, Hudes RS, Shepard D, et al. Fetal and ovarian radiation dose in patients undergoing gamma knife radiosurgery. Surg Neurol 2002;58(1): 32–41.
58. Nagayama K, Kurita H, Tonari A, et al. Radiosurgery for cerebral arteriovenous malformation during pregnancy: a case report focusing on fetal exposure to radiation. Asian J Neurosurg 2010;5(2):73–7.
59. He S, Mack WJ. Considering radiation exposure during diagnostic and therapeutic procedures for arteriovenous malformations in the setting of pregnancy. World Neurosurg 2014;81(1):22–4.
60. Pantelis E, Antypas C, Frassanito MC, et al. Radiation dose to the fetus during cyberKnife radiosurgery for a brain tumor in pregnancy. Phys Med 2016;32(1):237–41.
61. Pavlidis N, Pentheroudakis G. Metastatic involvement of placenta and foetus in pregnant women with cancer. Recent Results Cancer Res 2008;178: 183–94.

Thoracic Surgery in Early-Stage Small Cell Lung Cancer

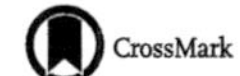

Matthew Low, MD[a], Sharon Ben-Or, MD[b,*]

KEYWORDS

• Early stage • Small cell lung cancer • Surgical treatment

KEY POINTS

- Patients with limited stage small cell lung cancer, stage I (T1-T2, N0) should be offered surgery as part of their treatment plan.
- Lobectomy is the surgery of choice in patients who can tolerate the procedure.
- Surgery with chemotherapy should be used because this can increase 5-year survival.

INTRODUCTION: NATURE OF THE PROBLEM

In 2017, approximately 222,500 Americans will be diagnosed with lung cancer. From these new cases, 10%–15% will be small cell lung cancer (SCLC).[1] Since the origin of its name and description in 1926, SCLC has been difficult to treat because of its aggressive nature and significant rate of recurrence (50%–80%).[2–4] Before World War II, surgery was the initial treatment of choice in patients amenable to resection, whereas radiation therapy was reserved for those with unresectable disease. However, in the 1960s and 1970s, advancements in radiotherapy[5,6] and chemotherapy[7,8] were shown to have similar survival rates when compared with surgical management.

A recent review article by Haddadin and Perry[9] accurately divides the historical course of SCLC into 3 intervals: (1) the characterization of SCLC (1920s–1950s); (2) advancements in staging and treatment—chemotherapy and radiation (1960s–1980s); and (3) a dormant period during which advancements appear to have stalled (1990s–current). During this lull in therapeutic progress, questions have arisen about whether or not surgery is still a viable treatment option for early-stage SCLC. In this article, the authors discuss the current literature on treatment of early-stage SCLC and whether surgery should be considered a viable treatment modality.

THERAPEUTIC OPTIONS AND SURGICAL TECHNIQUES

Epidemiology

The American Cancer Society estimates the incidence of lung cancer to reach 222,500 in 2017.[1] In 1993, SCLC represented 25% of all lung cancers; today SCLC represents 10%–15%.[1,10] This significant decrease is thought to be attributed to downward trends in smoking, because the overall risk of developing SCLC has been related to the quantity and length of time a patient has smoked.[11]

Most patients with SCLC will present with metastases or extensive stage disease, rendering most disease not amenable to surgical resection. Only 4% to 12% of patients have solitary pulmonary nodules that can be classified as very early-stage disease.[12] Many think this is a result of the

Disclosure: The authors have no commercial or financial conflicts to disclose.

[a] Department of Surgery, Greenville Health System, 701 Grove Road, 3rd Floor Support Tower, Greenville, SC 29605, USA; [b] Division of Thoracic Surgery, Department of Surgery, Greenville Memorial Hospital, 890 W Faris Road, Suite 320, Greenville, SC 29605, USA
* Corresponding author.
E-mail address: sben-or@ghs.org

Thorac Surg Clin 28 (2018) 9–14
https://doi.org/10.1016/j.thorsurg.2017.08.003

increased number of mutations involved in SCLC that involve downregulation of TP53 genes and histone modification.[13] Even patients with limited stage disease typically present with evidence of hilar, mediastinal, or supraclavicular nodal involvement, altering their clinical stage and negating their ability for resection.[14]

Staging of small cell lung cancer

Initially, the aggressive nature of SCLC earned its own staging system separate from the TNM staging system. The Veterans Administration Lung Cancer Study Group (VALSG) was the first to assign the designation of limited-stage (LS) and extensive stage (ES) disease. LS disease was defined as a tumor confined to 1 hemithorax, and primary tumor and regional lymph nodes encompassed in a safe radiation portal.[14] LS disease included left recurrent laryngeal nerve involvement, nonmalignant ipsilateral pleural effusions, and superior vena cava involvement. ES disease was defined as anything that could not be classified in this category.

In 1987, the International Association for the Study of Lung Cancer revised the VALSG system to adapt to the TNM staging system: LS disease included stages I to III and ES disease included stage IV.[15] The staging was again revised in 2007 in an effort to further stratify patients with LS disease.[16] The identification of subgroups of LS disease followed a retrospective study on 8000 patients with SCLC. This substantial review showed patients with mediastinal lymph node involvement (stage III) to have significantly worse 5-year survival than patients with N1 lymph node involvement (stage II) (13% vs 18%; $P = .003$).[16] The 5-year survival rate was also significantly different between patients with stage II and stage I disease (21% vs 38%; $P = .008$). The TNM system, however, is limited in that it requires mediastinal lymph node biopsies with pathology confirmation at the time of surgery; only 2% to 6% of patients with SCLC present at a stage that is amenable to surgical treatment.[14]

Both the VALSG and the TNM staging systems are used today. However, the National Comprehensive Cancer Network (NCCN) has provided formal definitions for LS and ES disease, as follows:

- LS: American Joint Committee on Cancer (AJCC) (7th edition) stage I to III (T any, N any, M0) that can be safely treated with definitive radiation doses. Excludes T3–4 due to multiple lung nodules or tumor/nodal volume too large to be encompassed in a tolerable radiation plan.
- ES: AJCC (7th edition) stage IV (T any, N any, M1a/b), or T3–4 due to multiple lung nodules or tumor/nodal volume too large to be encompassed in a tolerable radiation plan.[17]

Current overall 5-year survival rates for LS disease are 48% for stage I, 39% for stage II, and 15% for stage III, respectively.[18]

Small Cell Lung Cancer Treatment Options

In the 1950s, SCLC was designated as a separate entity from other types of lung cancer. As previously mentioned, surgery was the initial treatment modality for SCLC. However, in the late 1960s, the Medical Research Council demonstrated there to be no survival benefit at 5 years for patients who received surgery compared with those who received radiation therapy alone.[5] In fact, the patients who received radiation therapy alone were found to have an increased rate of survival at 2 years (10% vs 4%), 4 years (7% vs 3%), and 5 years (4% vs 1%).[5] This same group continued their research and published a 10-year follow-up study with similar results. They evaluated 144 patients with SCLC randomized to surgery ($n = 71$) and radiotherapy ($n = 73$).[6] There were no 10-year survivors in the surgery arm, but 3 patients remained in the radiotherapy arm. Following the statistically significant difference ($P = .04$) in mean survival between the surgery (199 days) and radiotherapy (330 days) treatment arms, radiation therapy replaced surgery as the preferred treatment modality for SCLC.

Over the next several decades (1960s–1980s), chemotherapy was also shown to be successful in treating SCLC. In 1962, Watson and Berg[7] demonstrated the benefit of nitrogen mustard in patients with SCLC. Several years later (1969), the Veterans Administration Hospitals evaluated cyclophosphamide, which also showed benefits in survival.[8] In 1984, Feld and colleagues[19] evaluated 153 patients with LS disease who were treated with chemotherapy (cyclophosphamide, doxorubicin, and vincristine), thoracic radiation, and prophylactic cranial irradiation. Approximately 52% of these patients achieved complete response.

In 1979, Sierocki and colleagues[20] revealed etoposide and cisplatin to be a viable treatment option (complete response rate: 52%). Since then, combination therapy with etoposide and cisplatin, along with radiotherapy, has remained the standard of care. During this exciting season of new chemotherapy agents, much promise was given for a possible cure, because SCLC continued to have good chemotherapeutic responses. However, for the last 35 years, there has been a lull in therapeutic advancement, with no significant improvement in patient outcomes or survival in phase 3 trials of new systemic chemotherapies.[21]

In 2005, Brock and colleagues[22] reviewed 1415 patients with SCLC treated at Johns Hopkins Medical Institutions between 1976 and 2002. During this timeframe, 82 patients (6%) underwent surgery with curative intent. The 5-year overall survival was 42%. However, the 5-year survival rate for patients who underwent surgery along with adjuvant, platinum-based chemotherapy was 86%. Brock and colleagues[22] also found patients who underwent lobectomies to have better survival than those with limited resections (50% vs 20%; $P = .03$). Because of the success of platinum-based chemotherapy and radiotherapy, and based on the results of Brock and colleagues and other recent studies, the question of whether surgery should be considered as an adjunct to treatment of early-stage disease is being asked once again.

CLINICAL OUTCOMES

Surgery versus Nonoperative Management

The introduction of surgical resection as part of a multimodality treatment of early-staged SCLC has been extensively studied. In 2004, Badzio and colleagues[23] evaluated surgery with adjuvant chemotherapy to definitive chemoradiation therapy in patients with LS disease. Mean survival for the operative and nonoperative groups was 22.3 months versus 11.2 months, respectively ($P<.001$). The 5-year survival showed a similar trend of 27% for the surgical group and 4% for the nonsurgical group. Recurrence occurred in 53% of surgical patients at a mean of 20.9 months, and in 86% of nonsurgical patients at 7 months ($P<.001$). These advantages, however, were not observed in patients with N2 disease.[23]

The benefits of resection over nonoperative treatment in early-stage disease were further supported in 2010 when Schreiber and colleagues[24] reported a significantly longer 5-year survival (34.6% vs 9.9%, $P<.001$) and mean survival (44.8 months vs 13.7 months, $P<.001$) in the surgery group than nonoperative group. In 2012, Weksler and colleagues[25] observed similar findings, reporting a mean survival of 34 months versus 16 months in the surgical and nonsurgical groups, respectively ($P<.001$).

In 2015, Takenaka and colleagues[26] compared patients who underwent resection with and without adjuvant chemotherapy and radiation therapy to a nonoperative treatment arm. This study looked at 5-year survival in each of these groups with respect to stage. A statistical difference in 5-year survival was only observed for stage I disease, which was 62% for the operative group and 25% for the nonoperative group ($P<.001$). For stage II disease, the difference was 33% versus 24% ($P = .95$), and for stage III disease, there was no survival advantage for surgical resection with both arms having a 5-year survival of 18%. The investigators concluded that the survival advantage of surgical resection is only seen in patients with stage I disease.[26]

Multiple medical societies have come to similar conclusions. The National Collaborating Centre for Cancer, the American College of Chest Physicians (ACCP), and the American Society of Clinical Oncology (ASCO) have each issued statements that surgical resection is superior to definitive chemoradiation therapy for patients with clinical stage I SCLC.[27–29]

Type of Surgery

The type of resection can play a key role in patient outcomes. During the study to evaluate operative versus nonoperative treatment of patients with LS SCLC, Schreiber and colleagues[24] further evaluated the surgical group in terms of resection type: lobectomy versus pneumonectomy versus sublobar resection. The median survival time was 40 months, 20 months, and 23 months, respectively ($P<.001$). Patients who underwent lobectomy for localized disease had a 52.6% 5-year survival rate.

In 2015, Stish and colleagues[30] evaluated the type of resection with respect to intrathoracic recurrence. They found a greater incidence of intrathoracic recurrence in patients undergoing a sublobar resection (hazard ratio, 3.5; $P = .01$). Therefore, the type of resection not only affects 5-year survival, it may also affect risk of recurrence.

Schreiber's and Stish's findings have been supported by multiple studies,[22,25,31–35] furthering SCLC, because it offers superior survival and a lower risk of local recurrence than sublobar resection (**Table 1**). Moreover, as of 2017, the NCCN recommends lobectomy as the preferred treatment of stage I SCLC.[17]

Standard of Care for Stage I Small Cell Lung Cancer

Multiple studies have shown patients with stage I SCLC to have improved survival when undergoing surgical resection with chemotherapy versus surgery alone.[22,32,36] In 2015, Combs and colleagues[32] examined 2476 patients who underwent surgery for SCLC. These patients were divided into 2 groups based on treatment type: surgery alone versus surgery with chemotherapy. Patients who underwent surgery with chemotherapy were associated with a decreased likelihood of death

Table 1
Summary of surgical studies evaluating 5-year survival by type of resection in limited stage small cell lung cancer

Study, Year	Study Design	N Surgery	5-y Survival by Resection Type Sublobar, %	Lobectomy, %
Brock et al,[22] 2005	R	82	20	50
Schreiber et al,[24] 2010	R	863	—	52.6
Varlotto et al,[31] 2011	R	584	28.5	47.4
Weksler et al,[25] 2012	R	895	18.70	30.10
Takei et al,[33] 2014	R	243	30.6	58.3
Stish et al,[30] 2015	R	54	15	48
Combs et al,[32] 2015	R	2476	40	21

Abbreviation: R, retrospective.

(hazard ratio, 0.53; confidence interval [CI] = 0.43–0.65; $P<.0001$). Five-year survival was also higher in patients with stage I SCLC who underwent surgery plus chemotherapy than in those who underwent surgery alone (51% vs 38%).

The debate, however, of whether adjuvant versus neoadjuvant chemotherapy is superior remains unresolved, because no study to date has shown adjuvant chemotherapy to significantly improve survival.[36] In addition, no studies have found significant advantage in the use of postoperative radiation for stage I disease.[24,31] The current recommendation from ASCO, ACCP, and NCCN is that all patients with stage I SCLC who undergo curative-intent surgical resection should also undergo platinum-based adjuvant chemotherapy.[17,28,29]

Future Directions

Current ASCO, NCCN, and ACCP guidelines recommend that surgical resection be considered only in patients with stage I SCLC.[17,28,29] Some recent studies, however, suggest that surgery may also have a role in patients presenting with N1 and N2 disease. In 2017, Yang and colleagues[34] compared patients with N1 disease who underwent surgical resection with adjuvant chemotherapy versus concurrent chemoradiation alone. Patients who underwent surgery plus chemotherapy were associated with improved overall survival (hazard ratio, 0.74; CI = 0.56–0.97) and 5-year survival (31.4% vs 26.3%, $P = .03$).

Granetzny and colleagues[37] evaluated patients with N0 disease who underwent surgical resection and patients with N2 disease who underwent surgical resection after neoadjuvant chemoradiation therapy. They found that patients with N2 disease who had complete histologic regression of their tumor burden in their lymph nodes had comparable median survival with the N0 patient group (N0: 31.3 months vs N2: 31.7 months). However, those with persistent N2 disease had worse survival (12.4 months). These results suggest that surgery should only be offered in patients who are successfully downstaged following chemoradiation therapy.

SUMMARY

Treatment of SCLC has had a tumultuous history—from surgical resection to definitive chemoradiation therapy to combined modality in certain patient populations. Currently, standard of care for stage I SCLC is surgical resection with chemotherapy, whereas those with stage II or stage III SCLC undergo definitive chemoradiation. However, some studies have suggested that the role of surgery may be expanded to stage II and stage III disease as part of multimodality treatment.

Based on the importance of lymph node status in treatment planning, invasive mediastinal staging is essential. Therefore, when looking at someone's LS disease, the true TNM staging needs to be evaluated. TNM staging is likely to play a larger role in the future, because most recent studies do not evaluate patients based on LS versus ES disease, but rather according to TNM staging.

As treatment of SCLC continues to evolve, and as research into this rare disease continues, surgical resection may play a greater role than current guidelines suggest.

REFERENCES

1. Cancer Facts & Figures 2016. American Cancer Society (ACS) website. Available at: https://www.cancer.org/cancer/small-cell-lung-cancer/detection-diagnosis-staging/survival-rates.html. Accessed April 26, 2017.
2. Barnard WG. The nature of the "oat-celled sarcoma" of the mediastinum. J Pathol Bacteriol 1926;29:241–4.

3. Goldstein SD, Yang SC. Role of surgery in small cell lung cancer. Surg Oncol Clin N Am 2011;20:769–77.
4. Shepard F, Ginsberg R, Patterson G, et al. Is there ever a role for salvage operations in limited small-cell lung cancer? Lung Cancer 1991;7:394.
5. Miller AB, Fox W, Tall R. Five-year follow up of the Medical Research Council comparative trial of surgery and radiotherapy for the primary treatment of small-celled or oat-celled carcinoma of the bronchus. Lancet 1969;294:501–5.
6. Fox W, Scadding J. Medical Research Council comparative trial of surgery and radiotherapy for primary treatment of small-celled or oat-celled carcinoma of bronchus, ten year follow up. Lancet 1973;302:63–5.
7. Watson WL, Berg JW. Oat cell lung cancer. Cancer 1962;15:759–68.
8. Green RA, Humphrey E, Close H, et al. Alkylating agents in bronchogenic carcinoma. Am J Med 1969;46:516–25.
9. Haddadin S, Perry MC. History of small-cell lung cancer. Clin Lung Cancer 2011;12:87–93.
10. Govindan R, Page N, Morgensztern D, et al. Changing epidemiology of small-cell lung cancer in the United States over the last 30 years: analysis of the surveillance, epidemiologic, and end results database. J Clin Oncol 2006;24:4539–44.
11. Brownson RC, Chang JC, Davis JR. Gender and histologic type variations in smoking-related risk of lung cancer. Epidemiology 1992;3:61–4.
12. Quoix E, Fraser R, Wolkove N, et al. Small cell lung cancer presenting as a solitary pulmonary nodule. Cancer 1990;66:577–82.
13. Peifer M, Fernandez-Cuesta L, Sos ML, et al. Integrative genome analyses identify key somatic driver mutations of small-cell lung cancer. Nat Genet 2012; 44:1104–10.
14. de Hoyos A, DeCamp MM. Surgery for small cell lung cancer. Thorac Surg Clin 2014;24:399–409.
15. Stahel RA, Ginsberg R, Havemann K, et al. Staging and prognostic factors in small cell lung cancer: a consensus report. Lung Cancer 1989;5:119–26.
16. Shepherd FA, Crowley J, Van Houtte P, et al. The International Association for the Study of Lung Cancer lung cancer staging project: proposals regarding the clinical staging of small cell lung cancer in the forthcoming (seventh) edition of the tumor, node, metastasis classification for lung cancer. J Thorac Oncol 2007;2:1067–77.
17. NCCN clinical practice guidelines in oncology. Small cell lung cancer. National Comprehensive Cancer Network website. Available at: https://www.nccn.org/professionals/physician_gls/pdf/sclc.pdf. Accessed April 26, 2017.
18. Vallières E, Shepherd FA, Crowley J, et al. The IASLC lung cancer staging project: proposals regarding the relevance of TNM in the pathologic staging of small cell lung cancer in the forthcoming (seventh) edition of the TNM classification for lung cancer. J Thorac Oncol 2009;4:1049–59.
19. Feld R, Evans WK, DeBoer G, et al. Combined modality induction therapy without maintenance chemotherapy for small cell carcinoma of the lung. J Clin Oncol 1984;2:294–304.
20. Sierocki J, Hilaris B, Hopfan S, et al. cis-Dichlorodiammineplatinum(II) and VP-16-213: an active induction regimen for small cell carcinoma of the lung. Cancer Treat Rep 1979;63:1593–7.
21. Oze I, Hotta K, Kiura K. Twenty-seven years of phase III trials for patients with extensive disease small-cell lung cancer: disappointing results. PLoS One 2009;4:e7835.
22. Brock MV, Hooker CM, Syphard JE, et al. Surgical resection of limited disease small cell lung cancer in the new era of platinum chemotherapy: its time has come. J Thorac Cardiovasc Surg 2005;129:64–72.
23. Badzio A, Kurowski K, Karnicka-Mlodkowska H, et al. A retrospective comparative study of surgery followed by chemotherapy vs nonsurgical management in limited-disease small cell lung cancer. Eur J Cardiothorac Surg 2004;26:183–8.
24. Schreiber D, Rineer J, Weedon J, et al. Survival outcomes with the use of surgery in limited-stage small cell lung cancer. Cancer 2010;116:1350–7.
25. Weksler B, Nason KS, Shende M, et al. Surgical resection should be considered for stage I and II small cell carcinoma of the lung. Ann Thorac Surg 2012;94:889–93.
26. Takenaka T, Takenoyama M, Inamasu E, et al. Role of surgical resection for patients with limited disease-small cell lung cancer. Lung Cancer 2015;88:52–6.
27. The diagnosis and treatment of lung cancer (update). National Collaborating Centre for Cancer website. Available at: https://www.nice.org.uk/guidance/cg121/evidence/full-guideline-181636957. Accessed on April 25, 2017.
28. Jett JR, Schild SE, Kesler KA, et al. Treatment of small cell lung cancer: diagnosis and management of lung cancer, 3rd ed: American College of Chest Physicians evidence-based clinical practice guidelines. Chest 2013;143:e400S–19S.
29. Rudin CM, Ismaila N, Hann CL, et al. Treatment of small-cell lung cancer: American Society of Clinical Oncology endorsement of the American College of Chest Physicians guideline. J Clin Oncol 2015;33:4106–11.
30. Stish BJ, Hallemeier CL, Olivier KR, et al. Long-term outcomes and patterns of failure after surgical resection of small-cell lung cancer. Clin Lung Cancer 2015;16:e67–73.
31. Varlotto JM, Recht A, Flickinger JC, et al. Lobectomy leads to optimal survival in early-stage small cell lung cancer: a retrospective analysis. J Thorac Cardiovasc Surg 2011;142:538–46.

32. Combs SE, Hancock JG, Boffa DJ, et al. Bolstering the case for lobectomy in stages I, II, and IIIA small-cell lung cancer using the National Cancer Data Base. J Thorac Oncol 2015;10:316–23.
33. Takei H, Kondo H, Miyaoka E, et al. Surgery for small cell lung cancer: a retrospective analysis of 243 patients from japanese lung cancer registry in 2004. J Thorac Oncol 2014;9:1140–5.
34. Yang CJ, Chan DY, Speicher PJ. Surgery vs optimal management for N1 small cell lung cancer. Ann Thorac Surg 2017;103:1767–72.
35. Ginsberg RJ, Rubinstein LV. Randomized trial of lobectomy versus limited resection for T1N0 non-small cell lung cancer. Lung Cancer Study Group. Ann Thorac Surg 1995;60:615–23.
36. Xu Y-J, Zheng H, Gao W, et al. Is neoadjuvant chemotherapy mandatory for limited-disease small-cell lung cancer? Interact Cardiovasc Thorac Surg 2014;19:887–93.
37. Granetzny A, Boseila A, Wagner W, et al. Surgery in the tri-modality treatment of small cell lung cancer. Stage-dependent survival. Eur J Cardiothorac Surg 2006;30:212–6.

Lung Cancer and Lung Transplantation

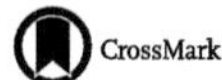

Timothy Brand, MD, Benjamin Haithcock, MD*

KEYWORDS

• Lung transplantation • Malignancy • Immunosuppression

KEY POINTS

- Lung transplantation remains a viable option for patients with endstage pulmonary disease.
- The issue of lung malignancy becomes an increasing concern.
- There have been concerns about the addition of immunosuppression increasing the risk of native lung malignancies in these patients. Despite removing the affected organ and replacing both lungs, the risk of lung malignancies still exists.
- Incidental evidence of malignancies may be identified in the explanted lungs of recipients.
- Regardless of the mode of entry, lung cancer affects the prognosis in these patients and diligence is required.

INTRODUCTION

Lung transplantation remains a viable option for patients with endstage pulmonary disease. According to the 2016 Annual Report of the International Society for Heart and Lung Transplantation (ISHLT), 55,795 adult lung transplants are entered into the ISHLT Registry. The median survival after primary lung transplantation for all indications is 5.7 years.[1] These patients have a substantial survival benefit and a dramatic improvement in their quality of life.

With improvements in selection criteria and perioperative management, these patients live longer. Because of this, as well as extended donor criteria, the issue of lung malignancy becomes an increasing concern. In the pretransplant population, these patients may have an increased risk of malignancy due to their smoking status or environmental exposure before being evaluated for transplant. This risk continues well into the posttransplant period, especially for individuals undergoing single lung transplant. The overall prevalence of malignancy is 5.1%, 18.2%, and 28.7% at 1, 5, and 10 years, respectively, after both single and double lung transplantation. Cause of death from all nonlymphoma malignancy is 0.1% (0–30 days), 3.0% (31 days to 1 year), 8.4% (>1–3 years), 11.8% (>3–years), 14.5% (>–years), and 13.7% (>10 years).[1]

There have been concerns about the addition of immunosuppression increasing the risk of native lung malignancies in these patients. In addition, despite removing the affected organ and replacing both lungs, the risk of lung malignancies still exists in these patients. Finally, incidental evidence of malignancies may be identified in the explanted lungs of recipients.

Regardless of the mode of entry, lung cancer affects the prognosis in these patients and diligence is required.

LUNG CANCER AS AN INDICATION FOR TRANSPLANT

Lung transplant for lung cancer was initially described in 1963 by Dr Hardy and colleagues[2]

Disclosures: The authors disclose no potential conflicts of interest.

Division of Cardiothoracic Surgery, Department of Surgery, University of North Carolina, Chapel Hill, NC, USA
* Corresponding author. University of North Carolina, 3040 Burnett Womack Building, CB 7065, Chapel Hill, NC 27599.
E-mail address: benjamin_haithcock@med.unc.edu

Thorac Surg Clin 28 (2018) 15–18
https://doi.org/10.1016/j.thorsurg.2017.09.003

from the University of Mississippi. This patient lived 17 days and died from complications related to renal failure and malnutrition. Currently, it is well established that patients with a history of malignancy within the past 5 years are not candidates for lung transplant.

There is a variant of bronchogenic carcinoma that may benefit from double lung transplant. Patients who have a subtype of bronchogenic carcinoma may be candidates for lung transplant. Initially called bronchioloalveolar carcinoma (BAC), it is characterized by a high incidence of intrapulmonary dissemination, whereas lymph node and extrathoracic metastasis is rare. In this context, lung transplantation could be an option in the treatment. BAC is now classified as either advanced multifocal (diffuse or pneumonic) adenocarcinoma in situ or minimally invasive adenocarcinoma of the lung.[3]

Patients with advanced multifocal adenocarcinoma may have a pneumonic-type lung adenocarcinoma that exhibits a diffuse consolidative pattern without bronchial obstruction. There are areas of both ground-glass appearance and solid consolidation, demonstrating the heterogeneous nature of this form of adenocarcinoma. Histologically, in addition to a lepidic predominant growth pattern, there may be areas of invasive components along with desmoplastic stroma. Alveolar spaces may fill with mucin, which would portend a poorer prognosis.[3]

These patients typically do not have nodal or distant metastasis. There is significant diffuse pulmonary involvement that renders the patient unresectable by thoracic oncologic standards, such as sublobar resection, lobectomy, or pneumonectomy, due to the bilateral nature of the spread. In addition, the rate of progression of lepidic predominant adenocarcinoma is slow. Therefore, some patients benefit from double lung transplant. This was initially described in 1997 by Dr Etienne and colleagues[4] for what was formerly known as BAC.

Because there has been a shift to mutational analysis for adenocarcinoma, a striking feature of mucinous adenocarcinoma is the absence of EGFR mutation but presence of KRAS mutation. It would make using a tyrosine kinase inhibitor ineffective in these patients but there is a growing use of drugs with a KRAS mutation.[5] Despite these studies, the 1-year survival for this population remains poor.[6]

In the patients with this variant of adenocarcinoma who are transplanted, the recurrence rate still exists. Some studies have demonstrated equivalent disease-free survival of noncancerous lung transplant subjects. In a study that used a questionnaire sent to 150 programs associated with the ISHLT registry, of the total of 8000 lung transplantations performed, 69 patients were found to have a bronchogenic carcinoma in the explanted lung with an incidence of 0.9%.[7]

Of these subjects, 26 were known to have multifocal (at the time) BAC. Nine subjects underwent single lung transplant. Four of these subjects died postoperatively due to primary graft failure (2), right ventricular failure (1), or cardiogenic shock (1). Seventeen subjects underwent double lung transplant with no postoperative deaths. Of the 22 subjects who survived surgery, 13 (59%) developed recurrence between 5 and 49 months after transplant (median of 12 months). Of these subjects, 9 died between 11 and 82 months posttransplant. Eleven of these recurrences developed in the transplanted lung. Overall survival at 5 and 10 years was 39% and 31%, respectively. Five-year recurrence-free survival was 35%

Another study used the United Network for Organ Sharing database to evaluate subjects undergoing lung transplantation with primary diagnosis of BAC or bronchogenic carcinoma between 1987 and 2010. Not included were subjects with incidentally discovered bronchogenic carcinoma. Twenty-nine out of 21,533 were identified to have BAC (0.13%). Double lung transplant was performed in 79% of BAC subjects. All explants were noted to have multilobar tumor involvement. Fifty-two percent (14) had pure BAC histology. Forty-one percent (11) had a focus of invasive or other features consistent with adenocarcinoma on a predominant background of BAC. Seven percent (2) had predominant adenocarcinoma, mucin production was noted in 11 tumors (41%), and papillary and acinar features were noted in 15% and 19% of invasive tumors, respectively. Of the 20 subjects whose lymph node specimens were evaluated, metastatic carcinoma was identified in 18.5% hilar nodes and 14.8% in mediastinal lymph nodes. A complete resection (R0) was achieved in 93% of the evaluated specimens. Graft survival was not statistically different between BAC and non-small cell lung cancer (NSCLC) subjects and noncancer transplant subjects at 5 years (44% and 47%) and at 10 years (19% and 24%). It was also identified that the evidence of invasive tumor or lymph node metastasis did not preclude the possibility of long-term survival. Presence of invasive cancer on histologic examination was associated with a trend toward decreased survival. From this study, subjects with advanced diffuse tumor have a high mortality rate associated with their disease process and median survival is approximately 1 year without treatment. The investigators suggest that a future study should involve a direct comparison of chemotherapy and lung transplant in comparable staged subjects to determine if a survival advantage exists with lung transplant. Finally, this study demonstrated that, despite common practice, lymph node metastasis did not significantly alter survival. Despite this, the investigators advocate for surgical mediastinal evaluation when feasible, in addition to standard staging imaging, while evaluating this patient population.[8]

LUNG CANCER IN THE TRANSPLANTED AND CONTRALATERAL NATIVE LUNG

The incidence of lung cancer in lung transplant recipients is higher than the general population. Risk factors include previous smoking and chronic immunosuppression after transplant.[9]

Immunosuppression reduces the natural antitumor immune response, predisposing transplant recipients to an increased risk for malignancies.[10] There has been an increase in the development of lung cancer in lung transplant recipients. This may be due to longer survival times for lung transplant recipients or an increase in the number of recipients with chronic obstructive pulmonary disease (COPD) and idiopathic pulmonary fibrosis because of the higher prevalence of smoking in this population.

In a study from Grewal and colleagues,[11] the prevalence of lung cancer after lung transplant was 1.9% (9 out of 462). Malignancy occurred more commonly in the single transplant versus double lung transplant population (2.7% vs 0.93%). In 7 of the subjects who received a single lung transplant, carcinoma was identified in the native lung in 5 subjects. In 2 subjects, the disease was identified to be metastatic. Cytogenic studies confirmed this to be recipient-derived. Two of the 9 subjects who developed malignancy after lung transplant received double lungs. In the 2 subjects who developed bronchogenic carcinoma, this occurred in the right mainstem bronchus in a subject with COPD. This was thought to be recipient-related. In the second subject, the malignancy derived from the right hilum. Cytogenic studies were unable to determine the etiologic factors of the tumor.

In another study, out of 633 lung transplant subjects, lung cancer was detected in 3.63% (23 subjects). Eighteen subjects were identified during follow-up: 12 cases in the native lung and 6 cases in the donor lung. The diagnosis was evident in the explanted lung in 5 subjects. The median time from transplantation to cancer diagnosis was 39.7 months. Survival at 1 year from diagnosis of lung cancer was 45.6%.[12]

INCIDENTAL FINDING OF LUNG CANCER IN THE EXPLANTED LUNG

Because of the etiologic factors of the patient's endstage lung disease, these patients are already at increased risk compared with the general population for lung malignancy. Therefore, during the time of explant, occult bronchogenic carcinomas may exist. The largest experience was a multicenter survey from 67 programs. Out of 8000 lung transplantation, 69 subjects were identified to have bronchogenic carcinoma. Out of these subjects, 43 were identified to be incidental at the time of transplant. The indications for transplant in these subjects were emphysema (26), idiopathic pulmonary fibrosis (11), scleroderma (2), sarcoidosis (2), silicosis (1), and hypersensitivity pneumonitis (1). The tumor (T) and node (N) stages (from the 5th edition of the AJCC Lung Cancer staging guidelines) of these subjects were T1N0 (19), T2N0 (3) T12N1 (12), and T12N2 (2). Multifocal BAC was confined to 1 lung in 6 subjects and to both lungs in 1 subject. Fourteen of the 22 subjects with stage I NSCLC were alive at 30 months. Five subjects with stage I died of recurrence within 12 months. Nine of the 14 subjects with stage II or II NSCLC died from recurrence after a median of 8 months. Three of the 7 subjects with incidentally identified BAC died from recurrence.[5]

In another study of 462 subjects, the incidence of finding an incidental lung nodule was 1.2% (6 out of 462). Five were in subjects with interstitial pulmonary fibrosis (IPF), 1 in a subject with sarcoidosis. This resulted in a prevalence of malignancy of 4.1% in interstitial lung disease (ILD) subjects and 4.2% in those transplanted for pulmonary fibrosis. All of the malignancies identified were for adenocarcinoma.[11] In these 6 subjects, 2 had early-stage disease (stage I) and, therefore, surgery was curative. One of these 2 subjects with early-stage I malignancy died 6 months after transplant of sepsis and kidney failure. Of the other 4 subjects, all had advanced disease with lymph node involvement. The study did not specify which lymph nodes were involved. Median survival for these 4 subjects was 16.5 months (range 7–25 months).

These data suggest in a certain group of patients, especially those with nodular disease as seen in IPF, it may be difficult to ascertain if an occult malignancy exists. When identified, lymph node and distant disease should be assessed to accurately stage the bronchogenic carcinoma. Treatment should consist of staged therapy for as long as the patient can tolerate the treatment. Currently, there are no compelling data to suggest augmenting immunosuppressive regiments.

SUMMARY

There continues to be concerns regarding donor shortage. Evolving technologies such has ex vivo lung preservation have assisted in increasing the donor pool. Despite this technology, donor availability remains a concern. Patients with certain forms of adenocarcinoma may benefit from lung transplantation. Further studies are important to clarify this challenging group of patients. In addition, newer chemotherapeutic agents may assist in treating this patient population before being evaluated for transplant.

Despite the timing of discovery, patients with stage I bronchogenic carcinoma experience excellent outcomes. Most patients with stage II or greater bronchogenic carcinoma develop recurrence and die within a year of transplant due to metastasis.

Most patients with multifocal BAC develop recurrence but this is limited to the transplanted lung and is slow-growing despite immunosuppressive therapy. Therefore, transplant remains an option in this group of patients.

Before evaluation, if there are concerns of malignancy, these patients should be appropriately staged, as with any patients with lung cancer. This includes PET–computed tomography (CT) scan and brain MRI to determine if extrathoracic disease exists. Surgical mediastinal lymph node evaluation should also be considered to adequately stage the disease. In addition, biopsy of the lung parenchyma will assist in proving which classification of adenocarcinoma exists. Previous reviews suggest N2 disease may impair survival. Frequent monitoring of the patient's malignancy with CT scan while on the wait list will improve patient selection. All of these cases should be discussed and evaluated in a multidisciplinary fashion.

REFERENCES

1. Yusen RD, Edwards LB, Dipchand AI, et al. The Registry of the International Society for Heart and Lung Transplantation: thirty-third adult lung and heart–lung transplant report—2016; focus theme: primary diagnostic indications for transplant. J Heart Lung Transplant 2016;35:1170–84.
2. Hardy JD, Webb WR, Dalton ML, et al. Lung homotransplantation in man. JAMA 1963;186:1065–74.
3. Travis WD, Brambilla E, Noguchi M, et al. International Association for the Study of Lung Cancer/American Thoracic Society/European Respiratory Society: international multidisciplinary classification of lung adenocarcinoma: executive summary. Proc Am Thorac Soc 2011;8:381–5.
4. Etienne B, Bertocchi M, Gamondes JP, et al. Successful double-lung transplantation for bronchioloalveolar carcinoma. Chest 1997;112:1423–4.
5. Finberg KE, Sequist LV, Joshi VA, et al. Mucinous differentiation correlates with absence of EGFR mutation and presence of KRAS mutation in lung adenocarcinomas with bronchioloalveolar features. J Mol Diagn 2007;9(3):320–6.
6. Cha YJ, Kim HR, Lee HJ, et al. Clinical course of stage IV invasive mucinous adenocarcinoma of the lung. Lung Cancer 2016;102:82–8.
7. de Perrot M, Chernenko S, Waddell TK, et al. Role of lung transplantation in the treatment of bronchogenic carcinomas for patients with end-stage pulmonary disease. J Clin Oncol 2004;22:4351–6.
8. Ahmad U, Wang Z, Bryant A, et al. Outcomes for lung transplantation for lung cancer in the United Network for Organ Sharing registry. Ann Thorac Surg 2012;94:934–41.
9. Penn I. Cancer in immunosuppressed patients. Transplant Proc 1984;16:492–4.
10. Ahmad M, Rees RC, Ali SA. Escape from immunotherapy: possible mechanisms that influence tumor regression/progression. Cancer Immunol Immunother 2004;53:844–54.
11. Grewal AS, Padera RF, Boukedes S, et al. Prevalence and outcome of lung cancer in lung transplant recipients. Resp Med 2015;109(3):427–33.
12. Perez-callejo D, Torrente M, Parejo C, et al. Lung cancer in lung transplantation: incidence and outcome. Postgrad Med J 2017 [pii:postgradmedj-2017-134868].

Lung Resection in the Postpneumonectomy Patient

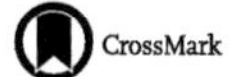

Megumi Asai, MD, Walter J. Scott, MD, FACS*

KEYWORDS

• Pneumonectomy • Lung cancer • Surgery • Recurrence • Metachronous cancer

KEY POINTS

- Pulmonary resection after pneumonectomy is a reasonable option in selected patients.
- Wedge resection for single peripheral metachronous disease has the best outcome with 5-year survival as high as 63%.
- Current and predicted postoperative cardiopulmonary reserve should be evaluated carefully.
- Stereotactic body radiotherapy is a promising alternative for inoperable patients.

INTRODUCTION

Pneumonectomy is commonly performed for resectable lung cancer and more rarely for trauma and selected benign diseases. Seven percent of 119,146 surgical resections performed for non–small cell lung cancer (NSCLC) from 2004 to 2009 were pneumonectomies.[1] After pneumonectomy for cancer, there is always a possibility of developing lesions in the contralateral lung. The risk of having recurrent carcinoma after complete resection of bronchogenic carcinoma is 2% to 5% per year,[2,3] and 1% to 5% for second primary lung carcinoma.[4,5] Although surgical resection is preferred for those synchronous or metachronous tumors, pulmonary resection after contralateral pneumonectomy is a challenging procedure that requires a thorough understanding of postpneumonectomy pathophysiology and the risk-benefit ratio of the procedure for that specific patient. Postpneumonectomy lung resection was initially reported in the 1950s; however, the number of cases in literature is still limited because of several restrictive factors.[6] Insufficient pulmonary reserve and advanced disease are the main limitations that prevent patients from undergoing postpneumonectomy lung resection. Grodzki and colleagues[7] reported that 82% of patients who developed lung cancer after pneumonectomy were refused surgery because of dissemination of the disease, central localization of the tumor, and functional contraindications. There is also a misconception on the part of some physicians that previous pneumonectomy is an absolute contraindication to additional lung resection even though satisfactory long-term survival can be achieved with acceptable morbidity and mortality for selected patients.[7–10]

The short-term and long-term outcomes after postpneumonectomy lung resection have improved over time.[11,12] Surveillance with computed tomography (CT) and follow-up PET detect second primary lung disease and metastatic disease in the early stage that may be amenable to resection. Careful patient selection, advances in anesthetic techniques including the adoption of lung protective strategies, improved postoperative management, and newer surgical techniques have all led to improved outcomes.

Disclosures: The authors disclose no potential conflicts of interest.
Financial Support: None.

Department of Thoracic Surgery, Abington Hospital-Jefferson Health, Price Medical Office Building, 1245 Highland Avenue, Suite 401, Abington, PA 19001, USA
* Corresponding author.
E-mail address: Walter.Scott@jefferson.edu

Thorac Surg Clin 28 (2018) 19–25
https://doi.org/10.1016/j.thorsurg.2017.08.004
1547-4127/18/

SELECTION OF PATIENTS FOR RESECTION

Appropriate selection of surgical candidates for subsequent lung resection after pneumonectomy is critical for a successful procedure. It requires multispecialty evaluation, especially focusing on the patients' functional status, cardiopulmonary reserve, tumor stage, and location.

Functional Status and Cardiopulmonary Evaluation

The American College of Chest Physicians recommends cardiovascular evaluation and spirometry to measure the forced expiratory volume in 1 second (FEV_1) and diffusing capacity for carbon monoxide (DLCO) before any pulmonary resection to predict postoperative morbidity and mortality.[13] It has been considered acceptable for surgical risk if predicted postoperative FEV_1 and DLCO are both more than 40%. When patients do not meet these criteria, the peak oxygen consumption greater than 10 mL/kg/min or 35% predicted may be adequate for major resection.

After pneumonectomy, FEV_1 and DLCO decrease from preoperative values by 34% to 41%, and 20%, respectively.[13] This negative impact on pulmonary reserve limits subsequent pulmonary resection significantly.

In addition, arterial blood gas analysis, echocardiography, and exercise testing are often performed to evaluate cardiopulmonary reserve. Pneumonectomy may cause elevation of total vascular resistance of the pulmonary circulation and an increase in the workload of the right ventricle.[14] Right heart dysfunction and pulmonary hypertension are considered absolute contraindications to surgical resection. Performance status is important to evaluate. Patients' comorbidities are also taken into consideration.

Assessment of Tumor Extent

Preoperative evaluation of a new lesion involves determining the stage and also the likelihood that the lesion represents a metastasis as opposed to a second primary.[7–9] Martini and Melamed[15] identified a second primary tumor when the cell type of the 2 lesions is different, the time interval between the 2 lesions exceeds 2 years, and the second tumor is in a different lobe or lung without common lymphatic metastases. When the cell type is the same in 2 lesions and the time interval to development of a second tumor is relatively short, it is less likely that a new nodule is a second primary.

Chest CT is used to assess the size, location, relation to adjunct structure, and characteristics of the lesion. Single wedge resection (wedge resection of only one nodule) has a better prognosis compared with more extensive surgery, such as multiple wedge resections, segmentectomy, or lobectomy after pneumonectomy.[9,16,17] Resections of small, single peripheral lesions are associated with the best outcomes.[7] Resections of central tumors or multiple lesions are not optimal, and alternative treatment should be considered. Judicious use of transthoracic or transbronchial biopsy may be considered in order to obtain a tissue diagnosis when resection is not planned. Grodzki and colleagues[7] used percutaneous biopsy in 83% of patients with a 13% rate of pneumothorax, which did not require intervention. This process may save patients from unnecessary surgery; however, sometimes it is nondiagnostic. Pneumothorax occurs after transbronchial lung biopsy in approximately 1% to 6% of cases,[18] while pneumothorax after percutaneous fine needle aspiration (FNA) occurs in 0% to 61% of cases with an intervention (chest drain) needed from 0% to 13% of the time.[19] Obviously pneumothorax can be life-threatening for a patient with a single lung. The clinician performing the biopsy should be prepared to place a percutaneous drain immediately should symptomatic pneumothorax occur. Bronchial lavage can retrieve a specimen for cytology with low risk of pneumothorax, but the diagnostic yield is low. Bronchoscopy is useful to identify any endobronchial invasion of the tumor.

Grodtzki and colleagues[7] noted decreased survival for patients undergoing postpneumonectomy lung resection who were found to have N2 disease compared with those who had only N0-N1 disease. Therefore, mediastinal lymphadenopathy should be evaluated by endobronchial ultrasound (EBUS)-guided FNA. Cervical mediastinoscopy can be performed, although it may be challenging given the previous surgical procedure, mediastinal shift after pneumonectomy, and any previous mediastinal radiation therapy. Postpneumonectomy patients with proven N2 lymph node metastases should generally not be offered lung resection. PET/CT should be considered for all patients to evaluate the likelihood of malignancy of a lung nodule, assess involvement of mediastinal lymph nodes, and look for distant metastasis. Mediastinal lymph nodes less than 10 mm on CT can be positive for metastasis on pathology, which correlate with poor survival rate.[7,8] The use of PET can save 1 in 5 patients with NSCLC from unnecessary surgery compared with conventional study alone.[20] The authors recommend brain MR in these patients if they have a previous history of lung cancer.

Postpneumonectomy lung resection is not limited to malignancy; however, the risk-benefit ratio should be carefully considered given the nature of the procedure.

SURGICAL TECHNIQUE

Perioperative management continues to improve. Lung protective ventilation has become standard for single-lung ventilation. There are more case reports about novel techniques of segmental lung isolation and high-frequency jet ventilation with combinations of thoracoscopic surgery and lung resections such as right middle lobectomies. Regardless of what technique is used, communication among surgical, anesthesia, and nursing staff is vital during the perioperative phase.

Anesthetic Management

A single lumen tube is used to ventilate the patient. Brief hyperventilation followed by intermittent apnea is often adequate to complete wedge resection, especially when an open procedure is planned. High-frequency jet ventilation and segmental lung isolation with bronchial blocker are occasionally used for both open and thoracoscopic procedures but are more advantageous for thoracoscopic procedures.[7,21–24] The use of extracorporeal membrane oxygenation and cardiopulmonary bypass has been reported but is rarely necessary.[25,26] Ventilation during operation should follow one-lung protective ventilation in order to avoid postoperative pulmonary complications. It is known that both high and low lung volume can cause alveolar damage and subsequent inflammatory response.[27,28] Tidal volume equal to or less than 6 mL per ideal body weight with positive end-expiratory pressure of at least 5 cm H_2O seems to improve outcomes.[27,29] Intermittent lung recruitment is also beneficial. Capnography and pulse oximeter are used for continuous respiratory monitoring. An arterial line may be placed for hemodynamic monitoring.

Postoperative pain control is very important to help respiration and decrease pulmonary complications. Patient-controlled analgesia and epidural analgesia are effective particularly after thoracotomy. Appropriate pain management should be planned before the surgery.

Surgical Procedure

Although sublobar resection may possess a higher risk of local recurrence compared with lobectomy in the long term, wedge resection and segmentectomy with hilar and mediastinal nodal evaluation are safe and effective alternatives for stage I NSCLC in high-risk patients.[30,31] A minimum 1-cm margin should be obtained for adequate oncologic resection and dissection, or sampling of at least 10 lymph nodes has been recommended for appropriate staging.[32] Previous studies have suggested that single wedge resection has better operative mortality and long-term survival compared with multiple wedge resections, segmentectomy, or lobectomy.[9,16,17] Lobectomy other than right middle lobe, which is considered equivalent to bi-segmentectomy, is especially high risk because of limited pulmonary reserve.[17] Although some have reported performing right middle lobe and other lobectomies with good outcomes in the postpneumonectomy setting,[21,24,33] this option needs to be considered very carefully.

Most procedures previously reported were performed through thoracotomy.[7–10,17,34,35] Median sternotomy is another option when mediastinal shift occurred after pneumonectomy and the lesion is located anteromedial. Recently, successful thoracoscopic wedge resection and lobectomy are reported with or without high-frequency jet ventilation and segmental lung isolation.[21–23] This approach may reduce postoperative pain and facilitate fast recovery. Another option for wedge resection of very superficial lesions is thoracoscopic wedge resection performed during standard ventilation with CO_2 insufflation into the pleural space. Insufflation provides sufficient space inside the chest for visualization with the thoracoscope even during ventilation (**Fig 1**).

OUTCOMES

There are a limited number of peer-reviewed case series available as well as sporadic case reports. Most recent series are summarized in **Table 1**. Five-year survival ranging from 37% to 60% with perioperative mortality of 0% to 29% has been

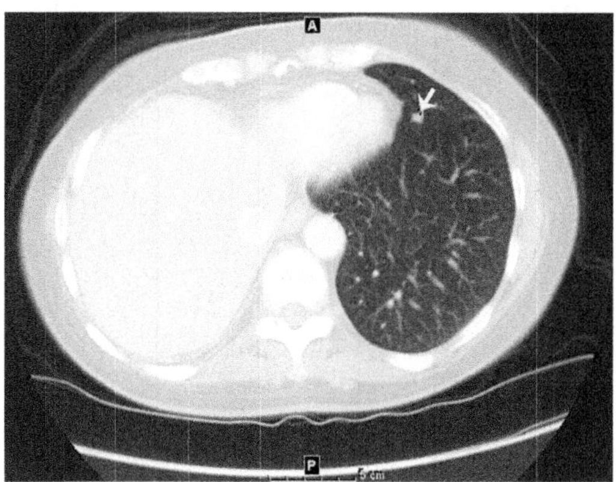

Fig. 1. CT image of a new superficial left lung nodule in a patient with a history of right completion pneumonectomy performed for recurrent atypical carcinoid tumor 3 years ago. This nodule was removed by video-assisted thoracoscopic surgery wedge resection using standard ventilation techniques while insufflating CO_2 at 8 cm H_2O pressure into the pleural space. *Arrow* points to lung nodule.

Table 1
Recent case series of pulmonary resection after pneumonectomy

Authors Name, Year	No. of Patients	Months to Recurrence, Mean (Range)	Type of Resections	Early Mortality (%)	Complications (%)	Overall 5-y Survival (%)	Metachronous 5-y Survival (%)
Kittle et al,[35] 1985	15	57 (4–192)	3 single wedges 5 multiple wedges	6.7	N/A	N/A	N/A
Levasseur et al,[16] 1992	7[a]	56 (24–204)	5 wedges 1 bi-segmentectomy 1 lobectomy	29	N/A	N/A	N/A
Westermann et al,[34] 1993	8	45 (14–135)	2 wedges 5 segmentectomies 1 lobectomy	12.5	25	N/A	N/A
Massard et al,[17] 1995	4	36 (12–71)	1 single wedge 1 segmentectomy 2 lobectomy	0	50	N/A	N/A
Spaggiari et al,[10] 1996	13	38[b] (9–90)	7 single wedges 2 multiple wedges 3 segmentectomies 1 thoracotomy only	0	31	46[c]	N/A
Donington et al,[9] 2002	24	23[b] (2–213)	14 single wedges 7 multiple wedges[d] 3 segmentectomy 1 lobectomy	8.3	44	40	50
Terzi et al,[8] 2004	14	35.5[b] (11–264)	11 single wedges[e] 2 double wedges 2 segmentectomies	0	21	37	45
Grodzki et al,[7] 2008	18	24 (4–106)	18 single wedges	0	N/A[f]	44	63[g]

Abbreviation: N/A, not available.
[a] Two of 9 cases in the report had pneumonectomy after lobectomy and no lung resection after the pneumonectomy and therefore were excluded from the table.
[b] Median.
[c] Estimated 3-y survival.
[d] One patient had 2 separate procedures, one single wedge resection and one multiple wedge resection.
[e] One patient had 2 separate single wedge resections.
[f] Seven complications are listed; however, no percentage of patients was available.
[g] Five-year survival of patients who had recurrence with more than 12 months interval.

reported. A high mortality in the earlier series was associated with lobectomy and segmentectomy. Overall outcomes have been improving, and this seems to be due to limited resection and better patient selection. Grodzki and colleagues[7] limited the procedure to single wedge resection and obtained overall 5-year survival of 44% with no perioperative mortality. Patients who developed second lung tumors with a greater than 1-year interval from pneumonectomy had longer 5-year survival (63%) in that study. Donington and colleagues[9] reviewed 24 patients and found mortality, complications, and 5-year survival of 0%, 28.5%, and 46% after single wedge resection, whereas they were 20%, 70%, and 25% after procedures requiring more than a single wedge (multiple wedge, segmentectomy, and lobectomy). Long-term survival is better for patients with a longer interval between pneumonectomy and the second surgery (5-year survival 0%–14% vs 45%–63%).[7–9] Positive N2 status adversely affects survival compared with N0 and N1 status.[7,8]

ALTERNATIVES TO SURGICAL MANAGEMENT

Stereotactic body radiotherapy (SBRT) seems to be promising for medically inoperable stage I NSCLC. It is reported to have a local control rate of more than 90% with great tolerance in high-risk patients.[36] Testolin and colleagues[37] reviewed 12 patients treated with SBRT for new tumor in the contralateral lung after pneumonectomy. All patients completed the treatment, and 2-year disease-free survival, overall survival, and disease-specific survival rates were 36.1%, 80%, and 88.9%, respectively. Senthi and colleagues[38] reported 27 patients who developed second primary NSCLC after pneumonectomy treated with radiotherapy. In this study, 20 patients had SBRT, 6 had hypofractionated radiotherapy, and 1 had conventional radiotherapy. They reported an overall 3-year survival of 63% with median survival of 39 months. Three-year local, regional, and distance recurrence were 8%, 10%, and 9%, respectively. SBRT is becoming a standard treatment of peripheral small peripheral NSCLC for inoperable patients. There was concern about increasing toxicity with central tumors; however, there are more recent reports supporting safety of SBRT for those lesions.[39,40]

Percutaneous radiofrequency ablation (RFA) therapy, on the other hand, is less promising with a high rate of complications and an inferior survival rate compared with SBRT. Recent studies[41,42] of RFA after pneumonectomy reported a rate of pneumothorax of 35% to 37% and 2-year survival of 59% to 71%. Although Yamauchi[43] reported a better survival and fewer complications, SBRT seems to be consistently better than ablation therapy.

The role of chemotherapy and conventional radiotherapy is limited because of the toxicity to a single lung and poor tolerance.

SUMMARY

Pulmonary resection after previous pneumonectomy is a reasonable option for select patients. Resections of single small peripheral metachronous tumors in patients with good cardiopulmonary reserve are associated with the best outcomes with a 5-year survival rate up to 63%. Physicians should carefully evaluate pulmonary reserve and cardiac function preoperatively. PET should be used with CT and brain MR to evaluate the extent of the tumor and to rule out metastases. Abnormal mediastinal nodes seen on imaging should be evaluated, ideally with EBUS. Patients with mediastinal (N2) lymph node metastases should not be offered resection in this setting. When the patient has an isolated lesion but is considered to be inoperable, SBRT is considered an alternative treatment.

REFERENCES

1. Rosen JE, Hancock JG, Kim AW, et al. Predictors of mortality after surgical management of lung cancer in the National Cancer Database. Ann Thorac Surg 2014;98(6):1953–60.
2. Pairolero PC, Williams DE, Bergstralh EJ, et al. Postsurgical stage I bronchogenic carcinoma: morbid implications of recurrent disease. Ann Thorac Surg 1984;38(4):331–8.
3. Fleisher AG, McElvaney G, Robinson CLN. Multiple primary bronchogenic carcinomas: treatment and follow-up. Ann Thorac Surg 1991;51:48–51.
4. Johnson BE. Second lung cancers in patients after treatment for an initial lung cancer. J Natl Cancer Inst 1998;90(18):1335–45.
5. Deschamps C, Pairolero PC, Trastek VF, et al. Multiple primary lung cancers. Results of surgical treatment. J Thorac Cardiovasc Surg 1990;99(5):769–77 [discussion: 777–8].
6. Rzepecki W. Is partial pulmonary resection after contralateral pneumonectomy in pulmonary tuberculosis feasible and indicated? Acta Med Pol 1960;1(3–4):259–67.
7. Grodzki T, Alchimowicz J, Kozak A, et al. Additional pulmonary resections after pneumonectomy: actual long-term survival and functional results. Eur J Cardiothorac Surg 2008;34(3):493–8.
8. Terzi A, Lonardoni A, Scanagatta P, et al. Lung resection for bronchogenic carcinoma after

pneumonectomy: a safe and worthwhile procedure. Eur J Cardiothorac Surg 2004;25(3):456–9.
9. Donington JS, Miller DL, Rowland CC, et al. Subsequent pulmonary resection for bronchogenic carcinoma after pneumonectomy. Ann Thorac Surg 2002;74(1):154–8 [discussion: 158–9].
10. Spaggiari L, Grunenwald D, Girard P, et al. Cancer resection on the residual lung after pneumonectomy for bronchogenic carcinoma. Ann Thorac Surg 1996;62(6):1598–602.
11. Mercier O, de Perrot M, Keshavjee S. Pulmonary resection after pneumonectomy. Thorac Surg Clin 2014;24(4):433–9.
12. Toufektzian L, Patris V, Potaris K, et al. Is it safe and worthwhile to perform pulmonary resection after contralateral pneumonectomy? Interact Cardiovasc Thorac Surg 2015;20(2):265–9.
13. Brunelli A, Kim AW, Berger KI, et al. Physiologic evaluation of the patient with lung cancer being considered for resectional surgery: diagnosis and management of lung cancer, 3rd ed: American College of Chest Physicians evidence-based clinical practice guidelines. Chest 2013;143(5 Suppl): e166S–90S.
14. Okada M, Ota T, Matsuda H, et al. Right ventricular dysfunction after major pulmonary resection. J Thorac Cardiovasc Surg 1994;108(3):503–11.
15. Martini N, Melamed M. Multiple primary lung cancers. J Thorac Cardiovasc Surg 1975;70:606–11.
16. Levasseur P, Regnard JF, Icard P, et al. Cancer surgery on a single residual lung. Eur J Cardiothorac Surg 1992;6(12):639–40 [discussion: 641].
17. Massard G, Wihlm JM, Morand G. Surgical management for metachronous bronchogenic cancer occurring after pneumonectomy. J Thorac Cardiovasc Surg 1995;109(3):597–600.
18. Izbicki G, Shitrit D, Yarmolovsky A, et al. Is routine chest radiography after transbronchial biopsy necessary?: A prospective study of 350 cases. Chest 2006;129:1561–4.
19. Covey AM, Gandhi R, Brody LA, et al. Factors associated with pneumothorax and pneumothorax requiring treatment after percutaneous lung biopsy in 443 consecutive patients. J Vasc Interv Radiol 2004;15(5):479–83.
20. van Tinteren H, Hoekstra OS, Smit EF, et al. Effectiveness of positron emission tomography in the preoperative assessment of patients with suspected non-small-cell lung cancer: the PLUS multicentre randomised trial. Lancet 2002;359(9315): 1388–93.
21. Fukui Y, Kohno T, Fujimori S, et al. Three-port thoracoscopic middle lobectomy in a patient after left pneumonectomy. Ann Thorac Surg 2015;99(4): 1422–5.
22. Walsh K, Park B, Amar D. Segmental lung isolation in a postpneumonectomy patient undergoing contralateral lung resection. J Cardiothorac Vasc Anesth 2016. https://doi.org/10.1053/j.jvca.2016.07.034.
23. Lohser J, McLean SR. Thoracoscopic wedge resection of the lung using high-frequency jet ventilation in a postpneumonectomy patient. A A Case Rep 2013; 1(2):39–41.
24. Nakanishi R, Hirai A, Muranaka K, et al. Successful video-assisted thoracic surgery lobectomy in a single-lung patient. Surg Laparosc Endosc Percutan Tech 2007;17(6):562–4.
25. Gillon SA, Toufektzian L, Harrison-Phipps K, et al. Perioperative extracorporeal membrane oxygenation to facilitate lung resection after contralateral pneumonectomy. Ann Thorac Surg 2016;101(3): e71–3.
26. Spaggiari L, Rusca M, Carbognani P, et al. Segmentectomy on a single lung by femorofemoral cardiopulmonary bypass. Ann Thorac Surg 1997;64(5): 1519.
27. Lohser J, Slinger P. Lung injury after one-lung ventilation: a review of the pathophysiologic mechanisms affecting the ventilated and the collapsed lung. Anesth Analg 2015;121(2):302–18.
28. Kozian A, Schilling T, Schütze H, et al. Ventilatory protective strategies during thoracic surgery: effects of alveolar recruitment maneuver and low-tidal volume ventilation on lung density distribution. Anesthesiology 2011;114(5):1025–35.
29. Liu Z, Liu X, Huang Y, et al. Intraoperative mechanical ventilation strategies in patients undergoing one-lung ventilation: a meta-analysis. Springerplus 2016;5(1):1251.
30. Donington J, Ferguson M, Mazzone P, et al. Thoracic Oncology Network of American College of Chest Physicians; Workforce on Evidence-Based Surgery of Society of Thoracic Surgeons. American College of Chest Physicians and Society of Thoracic Surgeons consensus statement for evaluation and management for high-risk patients with stage I non-small cell lung cancer. Chest 2012;142(6):1620–35.
31. Klapper JA, Hittinger SA, Denlinger CE. Alternatives to lobectomy for high-risk patients with early-stage non-small cell lung cancer. Ann Thorac Surg 2017; 103(4):1330–9.
32. Samayoa AX, Pezzi TA, Pezzi CM, et al. Rationale for minimum number of lymph nodes removed with non-small cell lung cancer resection: correlating the number of nodes removed with survival in 98,970 patients. Ann Surg Oncol 2016;23(Suppl 5):1005–11.
33. Falcoz PE, Assouad J, Le Pimpec-Barthes F, et al. Lobectomy for metachronous lung cancer after pneumonectomy. Eur J Cardiothorac Surg 2009; 35(2):373–4.
34. Westermann CJ, van Swieten HA, Brutel de la Rivière A, et al. Pulmonary resection after pneumonectomy in patients with bronchogenic carcinoma. J Thorac Cardiovasc Surg 1993;106(5):868–74.

35. Kittle CF, Faber LP, Jensik RJ, et al. Pulmonary resection in patients after pneumonectomy. Ann Thorac Surg 1985;40(3):294–9.
36. Maquilan G, Timmerman R. Stereotactic body radiation therapy for early-stage lung cancer. Cancer J 2016;22(4):274–9.
37. Testolin A, Favretto MS, Cora S, et al. Stereotactic body radiation therapy for a new lung cancer arising after pneumonectomy: dosimetric evaluation and pulmonary toxicity. Br J Radiol 2015;88(1055): 20150228.
38. Senthi S, Haasbeek CJ, Lagerwaard FJ, et al. Radiotherapy for a second primary lung cancer arising post-pneumonectomy: planning considerations and clinical outcomes. J Thorac Dis 2013; 5(2):116–22.
39. Lischalk JW, Malik RM, Collins SP, et al. Stereotactic body radiotherapy (SBRT) for high-risk central pulmonary metastases. Radiat Oncol 2016;11:28.
40. Rowe BP, Boffa DJ, Wilson LD, et al. Stereotactic body radiotherapy for central lung tumors. J Thorac Oncol 2012;7(9):1394–9.
41. Hess A, Palussière J, Goyers JF, et al. Pulmonary radiofrequency ablation in patients with a single lung: feasibility, efficacy, and tolerance. Radiology 2011; 258(2):635–42.
42. Sofocleous CT, May B, Petre EN, et al. Pulmonary thermal ablation in patients with prior pneumonectomy. AJR Am J Roentgenol 2011;196(5):W606–12.
43. Yamauchi Y. Percutaneous cryoablation for pulmonary nodules in the residual lung after pneumonectomy. Chest 2011;140(6):1633.

Thoracic Surgery Considerations in Obese Patients

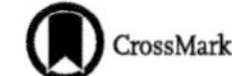

Douglas Z. Liou, MD[a], Mark F. Berry, MD[b,*]

KEYWORDS

• Obesity • Thoracic surgery • Comorbidities • Complications • Outcomes

KEY POINTS

- Obese patients pose special risks for thoracic surgery procedures because of physical body habitus and obesity-related comorbidities.
- Special intraoperative considerations are required when performing thoracic surgery on obese patients in order to minimize the risk of unanticipated adverse events.
- Postoperative care should be directed toward optimizing pain control, pulmonary hygiene, and ambulation.

INTRODUCTION

Obesity in the United States has been a growing epidemic for the past several decades. In 2014, 37.8% of adults 20 years of age and older were classified as obese (body mass index [BMI] ≥30), which was a steady increase from 22.9% in 1988[1] (**Fig. 1**). The percentage of adults with grade 3 obesity, or morbid obesity (BMI ≥40), more than doubled from 2.9% in 1988 to 7.6% in 2014. This increasing trend has been more dramatic over the last decade among women, with 40.4% categorized as obese.[2] In addition to gender, other factors associated with obesity include age, ethnicity, geographic location, and socioeconomic status.[3] The incidence of obesity-related diseases, such as hypertension, cardiovascular disease, diabetes mellitus (DM), and chronic kidney disease, have similarly increased over the same time span.[4] At present, approximately 1 in 10 adults in the United States are diagnosed with DM, with 90% to 95% of cases being type 2.[5] More recently, obstructive sleep apnea (OSA) has been recognized as a growing problem alongside the obesity epidemic given its important clinical associations with cardiovascular disease.[6] Higher BMI is also associated with increased mortality from all causes and therefore decreased life expectancy, particularly in the young adult population.[7,8] All of these obesity-related comorbidities have important implications regarding the risks associated with surgical interventions.

In addition to the direct deleterious health effects of obesity, other significant medical conditions in the spectrum of thoracic surgery diseases are more prevalent in obese patients compared with the general population. Several studies have shown a dose-dependent relationship between increasing BMI and symptoms of gastroesophageal reflux disease (GERD),[9,10] particularly in women.[11,12] A study by Che and colleagues[13] using upper gastrointestinal contrast studies on 181 morbidly obese patients revealed the presence of hiatal hernia in 37% of patients

Disclosures: There are no disclosures or potential conflicts of interest to report.

[a] Department of Cardiothoracic Surgery, Stanford University, Stanford, CA, USA; [b] Department of Cardiothoracic Surgery, Stanford University, 300 Pasteur Drive, Falk Cardiovascular Research Building, 2nd Floor, Stanford, CA 94305, USA
* Corresponding author.
E-mail address: berry037@stanford.edu

Thorac Surg Clin 28 (2018) 27–41
https://doi.org/10.1016/j.thorsurg.2017.09.004

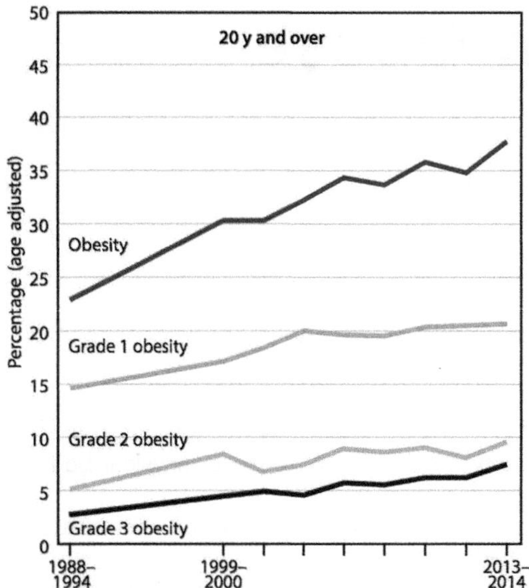

Fig. 1. Obesity trend in the United States for adults aged 20 years and older from 1988 to 2014. (*From* National Center for Health Statistics. Health, United States, 2016: with chartbook on long-term trends in health. Hyattsville (MD): 2017. p. 21. Available at: https://www.cdc.gov/nchs/data/hus/hus16.pdf.)

and GERD in nearly 40%. The high frequency of reflux disease also implies an increased incidence of Barrett esophagus in obese patients. Although data on this association have been mixed,[9,10,14] 2 pooled meta-analyses showed that increased BMI was associated with increased risk of esophageal adenocarcinoma.[10,15] Molecular and genetic studies also showed this relationship,[16,17] although the exact mechanism remains unclear and is likely multifactorial. Lung cancer is unusual in that it has consistently shown an inverse relationship with BMI.[18,19] The exception is a case-control study on patients who never smoked, or who had stopped smoking for at least 10 years, which found a positive relationship between BMI and lung cancer risk.[20] Nonetheless, the percentage of obese patients with lung cancer who present for major pulmonary resection has increased over the last several decades.[21] Many other cancers whose primary therapy is surgery have also been linked to obesity.[22] Overall, the prevalence of obesity alone makes it likely that thoracic surgeons will see obese patients routinely in their practices.

This article summarizes some of the key elements regarding the preoperative, intraoperative, and postoperative management of obese patients undergoing thoracic surgery. The importance of proper preoperative evaluation of obesity-related comorbidities is highlighted. Careful planning of the entire operation is discussed, which includes selection of the procedure, anesthesia and airway strategy, patient positioning in the operating room, and extubation plan. Postoperative pain control, pulmonary hygiene, and prevention of venous thromboembolic events are reviewed. In addition, literature on outcomes after surgical resection of lung and esophageal cancer in the obese population is presented.

PREOPERATIVE ASSESSMENT OF COMORBIDITIES AND RISK FACTORS FOR SURGERY

Obesity is associated with a variety of medical conditions that can affect the risk of undergoing major surgery and the occurrence of postoperative complications.[4,5,8] **Table 1** shows the accepted definitions of obesity based on BMI, and a list of important obesity-related comorbidities is presented in **Table 2**. Preoperative assessment of obese patients for thoracic surgery begins with a careful history and examination, with particular attention to signs or symptoms that could be associated with any of the conditions listed in **Table 2**. Findings from the history and examination should direct further preoperative testing.

Obesity is an independent risk factor for cardiovascular disease[23,24]; therefore, evaluation of underlying heart conditions should be a major focus of the preoperative assessment.[25] A thorough history should evaluate for the presence of hypertension, hyperlipidemia, DM, and other symptoms of coronary artery disease equivalents, including claudication or neurologic symptoms suggestive of transient ischemic attack. Dyspnea, fatigue, and lower extremity edema, although common and nonspecific in the obese population, should be noted given that increased BMI is associated with left ventricular diastolic dysfunction[26,27] and right ventricular dysfunction even in the absence

Table 1
Classification of body mass index

Classification	BMI (kg/m^2)
Underweight	<18.5
Normal	18.5–24.9
Overweight	25–29.9
Obese	≥30
Grade 1	30–34.9
Grade 2	35–39.9
Grade 3 (morbid obesity)	≥40
Grade 4	≥50
Grade 5	≥60

Table 2
Obesity-related comorbidities

Cardiac	Pulmonary
Hypertension	Restrictive lung disease
Hyperlipidemia	Obstructive sleep apnea
Coronary artery disease	Obesity hypoventilation syndrome
Cardiomyopathy	Pulmonary hypertension
Arrhythmias	Fatty liver disease
Heart failure	Osteoarthritis
DM/insulin resistance	Venous thromboembolism
Renal insufficiency	Stroke

of OSA.[28] Prior cardiac studies, such as echocardiography or stress test, should be reviewed if previously performed, along with the reasons why these tests were undertaken. Experience with prior surgeries should also be discussed, with a focus on any anesthesia or airway difficulties and postoperative pain management strategies. Medications, in particular β-blockers, anticoagulants, and antiplatelet agents, as well as lifestyle factors related to cardiovascular disease risk, such as cigarette smoking and exercise, should be documented. A strong family history of early cardiac disease should make the threshold to perform additional tests even lower. Routine preoperative blood work and a 12-lead electrocardiogram (ECG) should be obtained, whereas most potential thoracic surgery patients will already have had chest imaging with chest radiograph or computed tomography scan before their appointments.

Patients with signs and symptoms of heart failure or valvular disease require an echocardiogram to evaluate cardiac function. ECG findings of right ventricular hypertrophy, such as right-axis deviation and right bundle branch block, suggest pulmonary hypertension and also warrant obtaining an echocardiogram. Knowing whether pulmonary hypertension is present before thoracic surgery is particularly important considering that pulmonary hypertension can significantly affect a patient's ability to tolerate single-lung ventilation during surgery as well as a major lung resection. The body habitus of obese patients can make transthoracic echocardiogram technically challenging, and a poor or inadequate study should lead to a transesophageal approach. A left bundle branch block on ECG may indicate occult coronary artery disease and should be evaluated with an exercise or pharmacologic stress test, potentially followed by coronary angiogram and intervention. In addition, patients should be evaluated for the presence of the following 6 risk factors for perioperative cardiovascular morbidity according to the Revised Cardiac Risk Index[29]: (1) high-risk or major surgery, (2) history of ischemic heart disease, (3) history of congestive heart failure, (4) history of cerebrovascular disease, (5) preoperative treatment with insulin, and (6) preoperative serum creatinine level greater than 2.0 mg/dL. Based on the American College of Cardiology (ACC) and American Heart Association (AHA) joint guidelines, patients with 3 or more of these risk factors should undergo further noninvasive testing.[30] Considering that almost all thoracic surgery procedures qualify as major surgery, morbidly obese patients with any risk factor should be strongly considered for further testing.

Pulmonary physiology in obese patients has a restrictive lung disease pattern primarily caused by increased intra-abdominal pressure and decreased chest wall compliance from excess weight.[8,31] This pattern leads to lower static and dynamic lung volumes as well as increased work of breathing,[32,33] which have important clinical implications, particularly during anesthesia and the postoperative period. On induction, desaturation occurs more quickly because of increased airway resistance and atelectasis. Postoperatively, increased work of breathing following extubation combined with incisional pain and narcotic administration can lead to hypoxemia and respiratory failure.[31] Although little can be done to address the restrictive pulmonary mechanics preoperatively aside from weight loss, recognition of this problem is important for proper anesthesia planning and postoperative monitoring and management.

One of the most significant respiratory conditions associated with obesity is OSA. Approximately 70% of patients with OSA are obese, and the prevalence of this disorder among obese patients is around 40%.[33] OSA is characterized by inability of the pharyngeal musculature to maintain patency, with geometric alterations of the airway during the breathing cycle leading to intermittent upper airway obstruction. Increasing respiratory efforts to overcome the collapsed airway results in repetitive sleep arousal and profoundly fragmented sleep patterns.[4] The resulting chronic hypoxemia leads to pulmonary and systemic vasoconstriction, increased risk of cardiac and cerebral ischemia, and intrapulmonary shunting.[31] There is evidence that OSA is linked to cardiovascular disease, which further compounds the cardiac risks discussed earlier. Contributing factors include systemic hypertension caused by sympathetic activation from periods of hypoxia, a proinflammatory state related to chronic hypoxic stress, endothelial dysfunction caused by decreased availability of nitric oxide secondary to increased oxidative stress, frequent changes in intrathoracic pressure causing transmural gradients across the heart and aorta, and disruption of the normal circadian rhythm.[6] As with other respiratory alterations in the obese population, weight loss is the only durable solution. One study on OSA in morbidly obese patients showed that weight loss of about 15% of baseline body weight could substantially increase pharyngeal cross-sectional area and improve the severity of symptoms.[34] Obesity hypoventilation syndrome (OHS) is a related disorder characterized by hypercapnia ($Paco_2$ >45 mm Hg) and hypoxemia while awake, in contrast with OSA, which occurs only during sleep. The presence and severity of OHS is linearly related to BMI, occurring rarely in patients with BMI less than 30 but in 31% of patients with BMI greater than or equal to 35.[35] Screening for both OSA and OHS can be performed using the STOP-BANG (snore loudly, tired during the day, observed apnea episodes, high blood pressure, BMI >35, age >50 years, neck circumference >40 cm, male gender) questionnaire.[36]

A consequence of untreated OSA and OHS is the development of pulmonary hypertension, which can progress to cor pulmonale. Both OSA and OHS are independent risk factors for pulmonary hypertension, with OHS being associated with more severe pulmonary hypertension and a higher likelihood of right heart failure. Approximately 20% of patients with OSA develop pulmonary hypertension compared with 50% in patients with OHS.[37] From a surgical perspective, pulmonary hypertension is associated with higher risk of morbidity and mortality following noncardiac surgery, particularly in cases in which pulmonary hypertension is severe.[38,39] As discussed earlier, pulmonary hypertension can also significantly affect the ability of patients to tolerate single-lung ventilation as well as major lung resection if required. Thus, it is essential to investigate the presence and severity of pulmonary hypertension in patients with symptoms or risk factors, either with an echocardiogram or potentially right heart catheterization. Surgery may be safe in select patients with mild pulmonary hypertension,[40] but this should be considered carefully when deciding between surgery versus alternative treatment methods.

Another important comorbidity for surgical risk stratification among obese patients is DM.[1,5] Worse surgical outcomes in patients with DM are caused in large part by atherosclerotic and microangiopathic processes that compromise end-organ function, such as renal insufficiency and coronary artery disease. Patients with DM have 90% increased odds of myocardial ischemia after noncardiac surgery.[41] Diabetic vasculopathy also contributes to poor wound healing and infection.[42] A large meta-analysis showed that surgical site infection was increased by approximately 50% in patients with DM.[43] These potential adverse events are important to consider during the surgical evaluation and the perioperative period of obese diabetic patients.

Other obesity-related comorbidities that can affect surgical risk and perioperative decision making include fatty liver disease, reflux disease, osteoarthritis, and history of venous thromboembolism (VTE). Nonalcoholic fatty liver disease (NAFLD) has become increasingly common with the increasing obesity epidemic. The natural history of NAFLD involves progression to nonalcoholic steatohepatitis in about 45% of patients, and approximately one-third of those patients develop progressive fibrosis.[44] The risk of undergoing a major thoracic operation could be prohibitive in patients who have progressed to cirrhosis, and thoracic surgeons should look carefully for signs of liver dysfunction even if there is no documented history of liver disease. The high frequency of reflux disease in obese patients and the potential for aspiration during intubation requires preoperative assessment of severity in order to determine whether the patient should undergo rapid sequence induction and intubation. Obese patients with severe osteoarthritis should be considered for physical therapy evaluation preoperatively to determine their capacity for mobility after surgery. If mobility is significantly impaired, the risk of postoperative pneumonia and pressure ulcers may be prohibitive and surgery may not be appropriate. Patients with multiple VTE risk factors, such as supermorbid obesity (BMI $\geq$50), prior VTE, history of coagulopathy, OSA, or pulmonary hypertension, may benefit from routine duplex ultrasonography evaluations for lower extremity clots and even prophylactic inferior vena cava (IVC) filter placement, although data on this subject are heterogeneous and not conclusive.[45]

Perhaps the most important aspect of the preoperative evaluation is proper discussion and education of patients regarding the surgical procedure, risks, and reasonable expectations during the recovery period and beyond. Patients should be counseled before surgery about the importance of participating in physical activity and pulmonary hygiene postoperatively in order to minimize the chance of complications. Alternative treatments should be discussed if this does not seem feasible or the surgical risk is too high. Examples of this include stereotactic body radiation therapy instead of surgical resection for stage I lung cancers, endoscopic mucosal resection or ablation procedures instead of esophagectomy for early-stage esophageal cancers, definitive chemoradiation rather than resection of more advanced lung or esophageal cancers, and placement of a tunneled pleural catheter instead of video-assisted thoracoscopic surgery (VATS) pleurodesis for malignant pleural effusions. For some nonmalignant conditions, such as benign esophageal disease, it may be judicious to postpone surgery until adequate weight loss is achieved. Evaluation by a bariatric surgeon for a surgical weight loss procedure before thoracic surgery may be beneficial and optimal for patients in these scenarios. Case reports of combined giant paraesophageal hernia repair with a bariatric procedure, such as gastric bypass or sleeve gastrectomy, in morbidly obese patients have been published,[46,47] although the safety of this approach has yet to be proved. The ultimate goal during the preoperative visit is to collectively determine the best course of action to treat the patient's ailment in the safest possible way based on the individual risk profile.

GENERAL ANESTHESIA IN OBESE PATIENTS

One of the most treacherous aspects of thoracic surgery in obese patients is the administration of general anesthesia. Obesity-related cardiovascular comorbidities discussed earlier can potentially increase the risk of hemodynamic instability while under anesthesia. The distribution and metabolism of drugs in obese patients are different compared with patients with normal BMI, and therefore careful dosing and titration are necessary. Management of the airway can be especially perilous because of reduced apnea tolerance and challenging anatomy. Careful preparation involving both the anesthesiology and surgery teams is paramount to avoid a catastrophic adverse event, particularly during induction and intubation.

Patients with increased BMI have reduced functional residual capacity, increased intrapulmonary shunting caused by a predilection for atelectasis, decreased chest wall compliance, and increased airway resistance, all of which predispose to rapid desaturation on induction.[25,31,32,48] This risk is compounded by the potential for obese patients, particularly those with OSA, to have a narrowed pharyngeal space that can make mask ventilation and airway access difficult.[49,50] However, obesity alone is not always associated with difficult airway in the absence of other contributing factors.[51,52] As such, it is important to conduct a thorough assessment for each patient to determine their individual risks. This assessment begins with a review of prior surgeries to inquire about any anesthetic or airway difficulties. Access to previous medical records can provide insight as to the degree of difficulty and technique used for intubation. History and severity of OSA and GERD should be elucidated to gauge the risk of airway compromise and aspiration, respectively, following anesthesia induction.[48,49] Standard examination of the airway should be performed with particular attention to neck circumference and Mallampati score, given that these are known predictors of difficult intubation.[51,53] Following the complete evaluation, the anesthesiologist and surgeon should agree on an intubation plan. In patients who have features associated with difficult mask ventilation and intubation, such as massive central obesity, short and wide neck, severe OSA, and high Mallampati score, the use of awake fiberoptic technique and the unlikely but potential need for tracheostomy should be discussed with the patient before surgery. At the time of induction, the surgeon should be present and all equipment that may potentially be used should be immediately available in the operating room, including a rigid bronchoscope and a tracheostomy set. This equipment is rarely required, but failure to have it when needed may lead to a catastrophic event.

Proper patient positioning before induction is crucial. Preoxygenation in a head-up position, with either reverse Trendelenburg or semi-Fowler position, prolongs the duration of safe apnea by optimizing pulmonary mechanics and functional residual capacity.[49,54,55] Rapid sequence induction should be used in patients who are at increased risk for aspiration, such as those with symptomatic GERD.[56] It is important to confirm sufficient depth of anesthesia before attempting airway placement because instrumentation of the pharynx in the presence of light anesthesia can lead to aspiration. Intubation is best performed in the ramped position, in which the head and neck are elevated such that the external auditory meatus is horizontally aligned with the sternal notch.[48,57] If visualization is poor with a standard laryngoscope, videolaryngoscopy may be useful. With adequate positioning and preoxygenation along with a backup plan, most obese patients can be successfully intubated following induction. However, if there is any doubt regarding the ability to mask ventilate or intubate, awake fiberoptic intubation should be strongly considered.

If intubation attempts are unsuccessful, general principles of difficult airway management should be followed.[58] The determining factor between an emergent versus nonemergent situation is the ability to mask ventilate. If mask ventilation is adequate, alternative means of intubation can be attempted, such as the use of a bougie or fiberoptic intubation. Alternatively, the procedure can be aborted and the patient awoken. If mask ventilation is insufficient, placement of a supraglottic airway should be done emergently. If this is unsuccessful, a surgical airway should be performed. Surgeons should always be mindful that an extended-length tracheostomy tube may be necessary for obese patients in this situation.

One-lung ventilation (OLV) is often needed for thoracic surgery procedures and can be achieved with either a double-lumen tube or single-lumen tube followed by placement of a bronchial blocker. A small randomized study showed no advantage of one technique compared with the other in morbidly obese patients with respect to successful intubation and lung isolation.[59] Securing the airway is the first priority, therefore a single-lumen tube should be used if there is any safety concern. Once the airway is secure, lung isolation can be achieved either with a bronchial blocker or by exchanging the single-lumen tube for a double-lumen tube over a bougie.[60] There are few data regarding the optimal strategy for OLV in the obese population. Two small cases series published more than 30 years ago on morbidly obese patients undergoing transthoracic gastric stapling concluded that OLV is reasonably well tolerated,[61,62] possibly related to lateral positioning causing the panniculus to fall away from the body and allowing greater diaphragmatic excursion.[63] It is not clear whether pressure-control or volume-control ventilation is best; however, the general focus should be on using high enough peak inspiratory pressures to open up collapsed regions of the lung and positive end-expiratory pressure to keep alveoli open.[31] This technique may not be technically feasible in very large patients because of increased airway pressures. Patients with pulmonary hypertension may also show signs of hemodynamic instability, because single-lung ventilation leads to hypoxic vasoconstriction that can acutely worsen the pulmonary hypertension. Before an incision is made, patients with hypertension should undergo lung isolation and be closely observed during OLV to ensure they will tolerate the process.

One example of such a case from the authors' experience involved a 50-year-old man with a BMI of 50 who presented with biopsy-proven early-stage esophageal adenocarcinoma discovered when he was being evaluated for a bariatric surgical procedure. Ivor Lewis esophagectomy via laparotomy and thoracoscopy was planned. During lung isolation, he immediately became hypoxic and required ventilation of both lungs. He remained unable to tolerate OLV because of atelectasis and derecruitment despite various maneuvers, including continuous positive airway pressure, therefore the surgery was performed via thoracotomy with both lungs ventilated and short periods of apnea that allowed completion of the procedure. Postoperative radiographs showed significant atelectasis and he required mechanical ventilation for several days before he recovered (**Fig. 2**). Other notable events from his postoperative course related to his obesity included the development of ventilator-associated pneumonia and rhabdomyolysis with acute kidney injury thought to be caused by the long period of immobilization both during and after surgery, although he ultimately recovered very well.

Extubation immediately after surgery is desirable, particularly following pulmonary resection, because of the risk of bronchial stump disruption and pulmonary air leaks with positive pressure ventilation. However, similar to the initial intubation, an extubation plan should be discussed and agreed on by the anesthesiologist and surgeon before proceeding. Bronchoscopy may be necessary to clear the airway before extubating. The patient should be fully awake and following commands. Repositioning to the reverse Trendelenburg position before extubation is important in order to optimize ventilation and provide better airway access if reintubation is necessary.[49] Extubation over a bougie should be considered if the initial intubation was difficult. The threshold for postoperative monitoring in the intensive care unit should be low. All health care providers caring for these patients must be aware of how the airway was managed in the operating room should the need for reintubation arise. The authors recommend that all obese patients be monitored with continuous pulse oximetry and telemetry, at least during the immediate postoperative period. In addition, obese patients should be admitted to a room in direct view of the nursing station so that they can be monitored closely for any potential airway or respiratory issues.

OPERATIVE PLANNING AND CONSIDERATIONS

Performing surgery on obese patients poses unique challenges from a technical standpoint. Increased body mass can potentially limit visualization, instrument range of motion, and depth of reach within the body cavity, particularly in patients with massive central obesity. Several

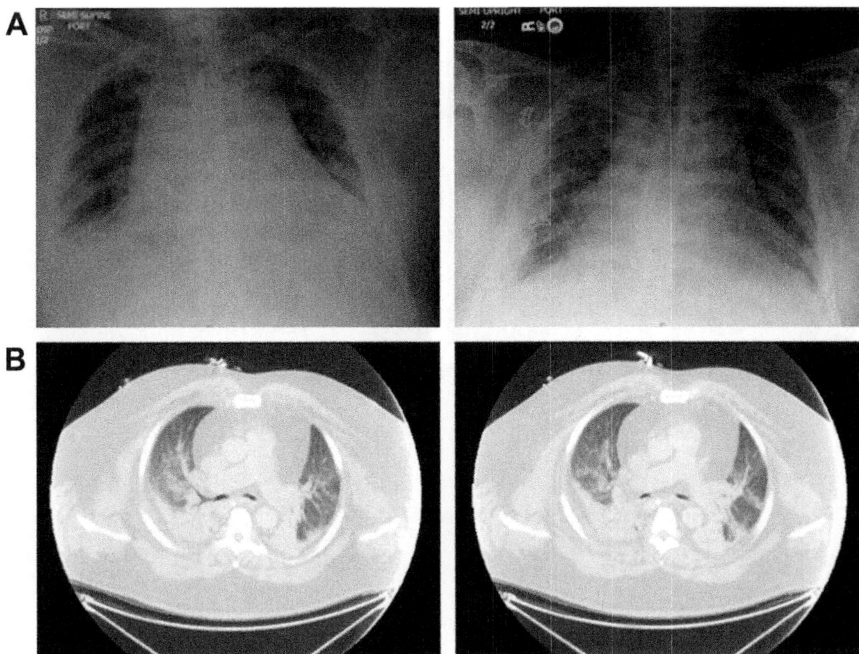

Fig. 2. A 50 year-old man with BMI of 50 who underwent Ivor Lewis esophagectomy for early-stage esophageal adenocarcinoma. (*A*) Chest radiographs from postoperative day 1 (*left*) showing low lung volumes and significant bibasilar atelectasis, which slowly improved over the course of 2 weeks (*right*). (*B*) Computed tomography chest showing bilateral consolidation caused by ventilator-associated pneumonia.

studies have shown increased operative time in obese patients undergoing lobectomy and esophagectomy.[64–66] As such, special considerations must be taken when planning an operation on obese patients, starting with the surgical approach.

In the current era of minimally invasive surgery, the authors recommend laparoscopy or thoracoscopy, with or without robotic assistance, as the first-line approach in all situations in which the operation can be conducted in a safe and complete manner. Over the last several decades, there has been an abundance of data showing the benefits of minimally invasive surgery compared with open surgery, including data on the obese population. In the general surgery literature, studies on gastric bypass,[67,68] ventral hernia repair,[69] and colorectal surgery[70] show decreased complication rates and hospital length of stay in obese patients undergoing laparoscopy compared with laparotomy. In particular, wound-related complications were fewer in all types of surgery when using a minimally invasive approach. Similar findings of decreased complication rates are seen in patients undergoing VATS versus thoracotomy for lung cancer resection,[71–74] although there is a lack of data comparing the two surgical approaches in obese patients. Nonetheless, the benefits of VATS compared with thoracotomy in the obese population can logically be extrapolated from existing data. The authors also think that, in most situations, a minimally invasive procedure is less technically and physically challenging for the surgeon, with better and easier visualization than an open approach.

Another situation that requires careful evaluation of the surgical approach involves lower esophageal disorders that can potentially be accessed from either the chest or the abdomen. An example of this is a distal esophageal diverticulum located just above the gastroesophageal junction (**Fig. 3**). In these scenarios, the authors prefer an abdominal approach if possible in order to avoid the need for OLV in an obese patient. However, it is imperative during the surgical planning to discuss the potential for conversion to thoracoscopy or thoracotomy. The anesthesiologist and operating room staff should be made aware of these possibilities so that appropriate preparations can be made. The operating room table should be set up with a beanbag ahead of time to allow lateral decubitus positioning, and a double-lumen tube should be place initially or a bronchial blocker should be readily available.

Positioning of obese patients in the operating room requires meticulous attention in order to avoid unnecessary injury to both the patient and operating room staff. Inadequate positioning not

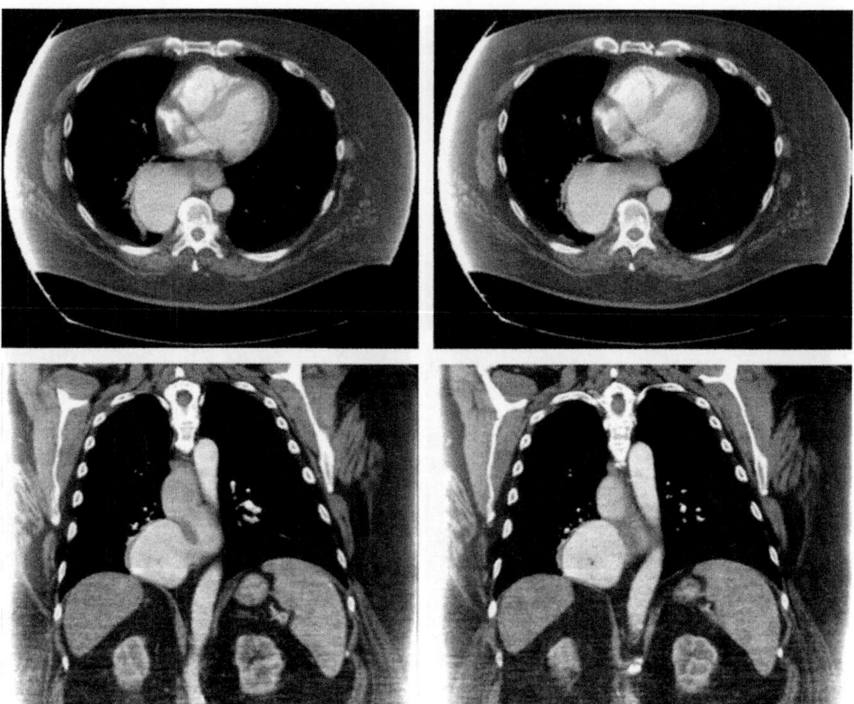

Fig. 3. A 63-year-old man with BMI of 49.4 who presented with dysphagia and was found to have a giant esophageal diverticulum approximately 5 cm above the gastroesophageal junction. Initial approach was robotic-assisted laparoscopy in order to avoid 1-lung ventilation; however, complete mobilization could not be achieved and conversion to right VATS was necessary. Ultimately, a successful minimally invasive esophageal diverticulectomy and myotomy was completed.

only has potential to harm the patient but also provides poor exposure, contributing to a more challenging operation. Transferring the patient from the gurney bed to operating room table is best accomplished using an inflatable transfer mattress to minimize lifting and straining. If not available, an adequate number of operating room personnel should assist to perform a safe transfer. Appropriate padding should be applied to all pressure points to avoid skin necrosis, including the iliac crests and bony prominences of the arms and legs. Padding is especially important when a prolonged procedure is anticipated, because studies have shown that irreversible tissue ischemia can occur after only 2 hours of 70 mm Hg applied pressure.[75] Similarly, rhabdomyolysis leading to acute renal failure can occur with prolonged immobilization, thus it is appropriate to check the creatine kinase level after a lengthy surgery to allow early diagnosis and treatment. If lateral decubitus position is required, the patient can be turned in the usual manner following intubation, again paying particular attention to pressure points. This position is generally tolerated well in obese patients, possibly because of the panniculus being displaced off the abdomen to allow better ventilation.[63,76] However, the panniculus should rest on the operating room table and not hang over the side because of the risk of pulling the patient off the table. Axillary support of appropriate size and position is essential in obese patients to avoid nerve injury from compression of the brachial plexus. VTE prophylaxis should be instituted in all obese patients given that they are high risk for thromboembolic events.[77,78]

POSTOPERATIVE MANAGEMENT

Postoperative care of obese thoracic surgery patients should focus on reducing the potential for complications for which obese patients may be at higher risk, which include pneumonia and VTE.[79] Avoiding these complications requires adequate pain control so that measures to maximize pulmonary hygiene and mobilization can begin early in the postoperative period. As such, a thoughtful pain control strategy is imperative to provide sufficient analgesia without causing oversedation and respiratory compromise. Use of regional or neuraxial anesthetic techniques along with nonopioid pain medications can reduce the amount of opioid required. In addition, given the predilection for wound infections in obese patients, particularly those with DM, close monitoring of the surgical incisions is important.

Pain management in obese patients should involve a multimodality approach. Although no formal recommendations exist specifically for obese patients undergoing thoracic surgery, clinical practice guidelines for general postoperative pain management advocate the use of multimodal therapy after thoracic surgery, including regional and neuraxial analgesia.[80] Guidelines for patients undergoing weight loss surgery and for patients with OSA also promote the use of central and peripheral nerve blocks as a means to minimize systemic opioid administration given the risks of respiratory depression in this patient population.[81,82] A randomized study comparing epidural analgesia with conventional opioids in obese patients undergoing laparotomy showed improved spirometric values in the epidural group.[83] Another notable finding was a significant and progressive decrease in all perioperative spirometry volumes based on increasing BMI. Alternatively, multiple studies have shown paravertebral blocks to be as effective as epidural blocks after thoracic surgery,[84–86] with the added benefit of fewer side effects, complications, and contraindications. However, one recent study noted that, when using local anesthetic alone rather than a mixture of local anesthetic and an opioid, epidural block was superior to paravertebral block after thoracotomy.[87] In addition to nerve blocks, the authors support the use of systemic nonopioid medications, such as acetaminophen or nonsteroidal antiinflammatory drugs, administered as scheduled doses as a means to provide baseline analgesia. Other adjuncts commonly used by the authors include patient-controlled analgesia systems during the first several days after surgery; medications for neuropathic pain, such as gabapentin; and transdermal patches containing local anesthetic. Patients should be asked about prior operations and pain management regimens that were effective. In challenging cases or in patients with a history of chronic pain, early and perhaps preoperative consultation with a pain specialist is appropriate.

Postoperative pneumonia is a complication that significantly influences both short-term and long-term outcomes after thoracic surgery.[88–92] Intuitively, obese patients are at higher risk of pulmonary complications given their restrictive lung physiology from excess weight[31,33] and increased incidence of atelectasis after general anesthesia,[93] which theoretically could lead to more difficulty in clearing pulmonary secretions and a higher chance of infection. However, data on this topic are contradictory, with some studies indicating increased risk of pneumonia after pulmonary resection and esophagectomy in obese patients[88,89,94,95] and other studies showing no difference.[96–100] The reasons for this discrepancy are likely related to heterogeneous study methods, data sets, and patient populations. The studies that did not show an increase in postoperative pneumonia may also reflect patient evaluation and care methods that avoided pneumonia. Despite this, there is little disagreement that postoperative pneumonia leads to worse outcomes, therefore the authors endorse an aggressive approach to optimizing pulmonary hygiene postoperatively. As mentioned previously, patients must be properly educated preoperatively so that they will be ready to participate in their own pulmonary care after surgery. Adequate pain control without oversedation is essential. A diligent nursing staff and respiratory therapy team can facilitate clearance of pulmonary secretions and encourage the use of incentive spirometer on a frequent basis. Patients who have poor clearance of secretions should be considered at high risk for aspiration, and precautions should be used as well as careful advancing of an oral diet postoperatively. For patients who struggle to clear their secretions despite all of these measures, therapeutic bronchoscopy should be considered early to avoid progression to respiratory failure. Obese patients should probably be counseled on this possibility during the discussion of the risks and benefits of their procedure before surgery. The same principles of airway management discussed earlier need to be considered when doing a postoperative bronchoscopy for toilet purposes in obese patients, including the need for appropriate sedation, analgesia, monitoring, and airway management.

Obesity is a risk factor for the development of VTE after surgery.[78,79] The American College of Chest Physicians guidelines recommend pharmacologic prophylaxis in all obese surgical patients unless contraindicated.[101] Because of the increased body mass and volume of distribution in obese patients, conventional prophylactic dosing may not be adequate and consultation with a pharmacist should be considered. Mechanical prophylaxis should also be instituted in all patients using sequential compression devices. Most importantly, it is imperative that patients mobilize early and frequently after surgery. Pain control must be optimized in order to facilitate frequent ambulation. If routine nursing care cannot adequately assist an obese thoracic surgery patient in getting out of bed and ambulating, a physical therapy team should evaluate the patient to assist in mobilization, document progress, and provide guidance on how to maximize mobility. Patients who are extremely high risk for VTE may benefit from a prophylactic IVC filter; however, data regarding the specific applications and benefits are not clear.[45] In one study using the National Inpatient Sample for patients undergoing bariatric surgery, in-hospital mortality in patients with documented deep vein thrombosis but no pulmonary embolus was significantly lower with an IVC filter compared with no IVC filter.[102]

As described earlier, obesity is strongly linked to DM, and more than 80% of type 2 DM cases worldwide can be attributed to obesity.[4] The significance of this in relation to surgery on obese patients is that DM is associated with impaired wound healing and subsequent infection.[42,103] Studies on patients undergoing coronary artery bypass surgery implicated obesity and DM as risk factors for superficial and deep wound infections.[104,105] The higher propensity for wound infections in this patient population does not necessarily prohibit surgery; however, diligent wound care and monitoring are required. In obese patients undergoing median sternotomy for mediastinal mass resection or other reasons, the use of a negative pressure wound dressing system after skin closure may be considered, because this has been shown to reduce the incidence of sternotomy wound infection in obese cardiac surgery patients.[106]

OUTCOMES IN LUNG AND ESOPHAGEAL CANCER

There is an abundance of data examining the association between BMI and outcomes after thoracic surgery for malignancies. Almost all of the literature indicates that obesity is not associated with increased morbidity or mortality after major pulmonary and esophageal resection.[96–99,107,108] Some studies did report increased complications in obese patients; however, in most instances the complications were categorized as minor and had no impact on perioperative mortality.[109–112] As previously outlined, obese patients have a higher predilection for significant comorbidities that can increase the risk of adverse events after surgery. However, obesity alone does not lead to worse outcomes when adjusting for these variables.[94,113] The findings that obesity does not lead to worse outcomes likely reflects general good preoperative evaluation and perioperative care that minimizes complications. Importantly, obesity should be not a contraindication to thoracic surgery intervention as long as careful planning and care are used.

Another interesting finding with regard to BMI and thoracic oncology is that underweight patients (BMI <18.5) have worse survival after surgical resection compared with patients with normal or increased BMI.[95,97] Investigators speculate that low BMI may be a surrogate measure for poor nutritional status in patients with cancer, which indicates a more aggressive tumor phenotype.[95,114] One study using the Society of Thoracic Surgeons General Thoracic Surgery Database found that both underweight and morbidly obese patients had increased risk of complications, whereas being overweight or moderately obese seemed to be protective after adjusting for confounders.[115] This so-called obesity paradox has been published on extensively throughout the surgical literature but the exact mechanism remains unclear.[103,116] Overall, the evidence again consistently shows that surgery can be accomplished safely in the setting of obesity, and therefore obese patients should not be judged as poor candidates for major thoracic procedures strictly based on BMI.

SUMMARY

Thoracic surgery in obese patients poses practical challenges for a variety of reasons. Many obesity-related cardiopulmonary comorbidities increase the risk of undergoing any invasive procedure, let alone a major thoracic surgical intervention. A thorough preoperative evaluation is critical to identify potential pitfalls and minimize the occurrence of avoidable adverse events. During general anesthesia, management of the airway must be meticulously planned and coordinated between the surgeon and anesthesiologist. A minimally invasive surgical approach should be considered if technically possible. Care of obese patients after surgery is centered on adequate pain control using a multimodality approach, aggressive pulmonary hygiene, and frequent ambulation. Proper patient education during the preoperative visit sets reasonable expectations for the operation and optimizes the chance of patients participating in their own postoperative care. Outcomes of obese patients undergoing major pulmonary and esophageal resection are generally equivalent to outcomes in nonobese patients who have similar comorbidities. Thus, obesity alone should not be prohibitive for major thoracic surgery.

REFERENCES

1. National Center for Health Statistics. Health, United States, 2016: with chartbook on long-term trends in health. Hyattsville (MD): 2017. Available at: https://www.cdc.gov/nchs/data/hus/hus16.pdf.

2. Flegal KM, Kruszon-Moran D, Carroll MD, et al. Trends in obesity among adults in the United States, 2005 to 2014. JAMA 2016;315(21):2284–91.
3. Wang Y, Beydoun MA. The obesity epidemic in the United States–gender, age, socioeconomic, racial/ethnic, and geographic characteristics: a systematic review and meta-regression analysis. Epidemiol Rev 2007;29:6–28.
4. Caterson ID, Hubbard V, Bray GA, et al. Prevention Conference VII: obesity, a worldwide epidemic related to heart disease and stroke: group III: worldwide comorbidities of obesity. Circulation 2004;110(18):e476–83.
5. Bhupathiraju SN, Hu FB. Epidemiology of obesity and diabetes and their cardiovascular complications. Circ Res 2016;118(11):1723–35.
6. Sharma N, Lee J, Youssef I, et al. Obesity, cardiovascular disease and sleep disorders: insights into the rising epidemic. J Sleep Disord Ther 2017;6(1) [pii:260].
7. Stevens J, Cai J, Pamuk ER, et al. The effect of age on the association between body-mass index and mortality. N Engl J Med 1998;338(1):1–7.
8. Haslam DW, James WP. Obesity. Lancet 2005;366(9492):1197–209.
9. El-Serag H. The association between obesity and GERD: a review of the epidemiological evidence. Dig Dis Sci 2008;53(9):2307–12.
10. Hampel H, Abraham NS, El-Serag HB. Meta-analysis: obesity and the risk for gastroesophageal reflux disease and its complications. Ann Intern Med 2005;143(3):199–211.
11. Jacobson BC, Somers SC, Fuchs CS, et al. Body-mass index and symptoms of gastroesophageal reflux in women. N Engl J Med 2006;354(22):2340–8.
12. Nilsson M, Johnsen R, Ye W, et al. Obesity and estrogen as risk factors for gastroesophageal reflux symptoms. JAMA 2003;290(1):66–72.
13. Che F, Nguyen B, Cohen A, et al. Prevalence of hiatal hernia in the morbidly obese. Surg Obes Relat Dis 2013;9(6):920–4.
14. Corley DA, Kubo A, Levin TR, et al. Abdominal obesity and body mass index as risk factors for Barrett's esophagus. Gastroenterology 2007;133(1):34–41.
15. Kubo A, Corley DA. Body mass index and adenocarcinomas of the esophagus or gastric cardia: a systematic review and meta-analysis. Cancer Epidemiol Biomarkers Prev 2006;15(5):872–8.
16. Chen Q, Zhuang H, Liu Y. The association between obesity factor and esophageal caner. J Gastrointest Oncol 2012;3(3):226–31.
17. Thrift AP, Shaheen NJ, Gammon MD, et al. Obesity and risk of esophageal adenocarcinoma and Barrett's esophagus: a Mendelian randomization study. J Natl Cancer Inst 2014;106(11) [pii:dju252].
18. Duan P, Hu C, Quan C, et al. Body mass index and risk of lung cancer: systematic review and dose-response meta-analysis. Sci Rep 2015;5:16938.
19. Yang Y, Dong J, Sun K, et al. Obesity and incidence of lung cancer: a meta-analysis. Int J Cancer 2013;132(5):1162–9.
20. Rauscher GH, Mayne ST, Janerich DT. Relation between body mass index and lung cancer risk in men and women never and former smokers. Am J Epidemiol 2000;152(6):506–13.
21. Ferguson MK, Vigneswaran WT. Changes in patient presentation and outcomes for major lung resection over three decades. Eur J Cardiothorac Surg 2008;33(3):497–501.
22. Arnold M, Leitzmann M, Freisling H, et al. Obesity and cancer: an update of the global impact. Cancer Epidemiol 2016;41:8–15.
23. Hubert HB, Feinleib M, McNamara PM, et al. Obesity as an independent risk factor for cardiovascular disease: a 26-year follow-up of participants in the Framingham Heart Study. Circulation 1983;67(5):968–77.
24. Poirier P, Giles TD, Bray GA, et al. Obesity and cardiovascular disease: pathophysiology, evaluation, and effect of weight loss: an update of the 1997 American Heart Association Scientific Statement on Obesity and Heart Disease from the Obesity Committee of the Council on Nutrition, Physical Activity, and Metabolism. Circulation 2006;113(6):898–918.
25. Poirier P, Alpert MA, Fleisher LA, et al. Cardiovascular evaluation and management of severely obese patients undergoing surgery: a science advisory from the American Heart Association. Circulation 2009;120(1):86–95.
26. Russo C, Jin Z, Homma S, et al. Effect of obesity and overweight on left ventricular diastolic function: a community-based study in an elderly cohort. J Am Coll Cardiol 2011;57(12):1368–74.
27. Sidana J, Aronow WS, Ravipati G, et al. Prevalence of moderate or severe left ventricular diastolic dysfunction in obese persons with obstructive sleep apnea. Cardiology 2005;104(2):107–9.
28. Wong CY, O'Moore-Sullivan T, Leano R, et al. Association of subclinical right ventricular dysfunction with obesity. J Am Coll Cardiol 2006;47(3):611–6.
29. Lee TH, Marcantonio ER, Mangione CM, et al. Derivation and prospective validation of a simple index for prediction of cardiac risk of major noncardiac surgery. Circulation 1999;100(10):1043–9.
30. Fleisher LA, Beckman JA, Brown KA, et al. ACC/AHA 2007 guidelines on perioperative cardiovascular evaluation and care for noncardiac surgery: a report of the American College of Cardiology/American Heart Association Task Force on Practice

Guidelines (Writing Committee to Revise the 2002 Guidelines on Perioperative Cardiovascular Evaluation for Noncardiac Surgery) developed in collaboration with the American Society of Echocardiography, American Society of Nuclear Cardiology, Heart Rhythm Society, Society of Cardiovascular Anesthesiologists, Society for Cardiovascular Angiography and Interventions, Society for Vascular Medicine and Biology, and Society for Vascular Surgery. J Am Coll Cardiol 2007; 50(17):e159–241.

31. Pedoto A. Lung physiology and obesity: anesthetic implications for thoracic procedures. Anesthesiol Res Pract 2012;2012:154208.
32. Malhotra A, Hillman D. Obesity and the lung: 3 obesity, respiration and intensive care. Thorax 2008;63(10):925–31.
33. Poulain M, Doucet M, Major GC, et al. The effect of obesity on chronic respiratory diseases: pathophysiology and therapeutic strategies. CMAJ 2006;174(9):1293–9.
34. Busetto L, Enzi G, Inelmen EM, et al. Obstructive sleep apnea syndrome in morbid obesity: effects of intragastric balloon. Chest 2005;128(2):618–23.
35. Nowbar S, Burkart KM, Gonzales R, et al. Obesity-associated hypoventilation in hospitalized patients: prevalence, effects, and outcome. Am J Med 2004; 116(1):1–7.
36. Chung F, Yegneswaran B, Liao P, et al. STOP questionnaire: a tool to screen patients for obstructive sleep apnea. Anesthesiology 2008; 108(5):812–21.
37. Friedman SE, Andrus BW. Obesity and pulmonary hypertension: a review of pathophysiologic mechanisms. J Obes 2012;2012:505274.
38. Ramakrishna G, Sprung J, Ravi BS, et al. Impact of pulmonary hypertension on the outcomes of noncardiac surgery: predictors of perioperative morbidity and mortality. J Am Coll Cardiol 2005; 45(10):1691–9.
39. Kreider ME, Hansen-Flaschen J, Ahmad NN, et al. Complications of video-assisted thoracoscopic lung biopsy in patients with interstitial lung disease. Ann Thorac Surg 2007;83(3):1140–4.
40. Wei B, D'Amico T, Samad Z, et al. The impact of pulmonary hypertension on morbidity and mortality following major lung resection. Eur J Cardiothorac Surg 2014;45(6):1028–33.
41. Hollenberg M, Mangano DT, Browner WS, et al. Predictors of postoperative myocardial ischemia in patients undergoing noncardiac surgery The Study of Perioperative Ischemia Research Group. JAMA 1992;268(2):205–9.
42. Baltzis D, Eleftheriadou I, Veves A. Pathogenesis and treatment of impaired wound healing in diabetes mellitus: new insights. Adv Ther 2014;31(8): 817–36.
43. Martin ET, Kaye KS, Knott C, et al. Diabetes and risk of surgical site infection: a systematic review and meta-analysis. Infect Control Hosp Epidemiol 2016;37(1):88–99.
44. Satapathy SK, Sanyal AJ. Epidemiology and natural history of nonalcoholic fatty liver disease. Semin Liver Dis 2015;35(3):221–35.
45. Rowland SP, Dharmarajah B, Moore HM, et al. Inferior vena cava filters for prevention of venous thromboembolism in obese patients undergoing bariatric surgery: a systematic review. Ann Surg 2015;261(1):35–45.
46. Patel AD, Lin E, Lytle NW, et al. Combining laparoscopic giant paraesophageal hernia repair with sleeve gastrectomy in obese patients. Surg Endosc 2015;29(5):1115–22.
47. Kasotakis G, Mittal SK, Sudan R. Combined treatment of symptomatic massive paraesophageal hernia in the morbidly obese. JSLS 2011;15(2): 188–92.
48. Kristensen MS. Airway management and morbid obesity. Eur J Anaesthesiol 2010;27(11):923–7.
49. Lohser J, Kulkarni V, Brodsky JB. Anesthesia for thoracic surgery in morbidly obese patients. Curr Opin Anaesthesiol 2007;20(1):10–4.
50. Kheterpal S, Han R, Tremper KK, et al. Incidence and predictors of difficult and impossible mask ventilation. Anesthesiology 2006;105(5): 885–91.
51. Brodsky JB, Lemmens HJ, Brock-Utne JG, et al. Morbid obesity and tracheal intubation. Anesth Analg 2002;94(3):732–6.
52. el-Ganzouri AR, McCarthy RJ, Tuman KJ, et al. Preoperative airway assessment: predictive value of a multivariate risk index. Anesth Analg 1996;82(6): 1197–204.
53. Gonzalez H, Minville V, Delanoue K, et al. The importance of increased neck circumference to intubation difficulties in obese patients. Anesth Analg 2008;106(4):1132–6.
54. Dixon BJ, Dixon JB, Carden JR, et al. Preoxygenation is more effective in the 25 degrees head-up position than in the supine position in severely obese patients: a randomized controlled study. Anesthesiology 2005;102(6): 1110–5 [discussion: 5A].
55. Boyce JR, Ness T, Castroman P, et al. A preliminary study of the optimal anesthesia positioning for the morbidly obese patient. Obes Surg 2003;13(1):4–9.
56. Freid EB. The rapid sequence induction revisited: obesity and sleep apnea syndrome. Anesthesiol Clin North America 2005;23(3):551–64, viii.
57. Collins JS, Lemmens HJ, Brodsky JB, et al. Laryngoscopy and morbid obesity: a comparison of the "sniff" and "ramped" positions. Obes Surg 2004; 14(9):1171–5.

58. Apfelbaum JL, Hagberg CA, Caplan RA, et al. Practice guidelines for management of the difficult airway: an updated report by the American Society of Anesthesiologists Task Force on Management of the Difficult Airway. Anesthesiology 2013;118(2):251–70.
59. Campos JH, Hallam EA, Ueda K. Lung isolation in the morbidly obese patient: a comparison of a left-sided double-lumen tracheal tube with the ArndtÆ wire-guided blocker. Br J Anaesth 2012;109(4):630–5.
60. Campos JH, Ueda K. Lung separation in the morbidly obese patient. Anesthesiol Res Pract 2012;2012:207598.
61. Oakes DD, Cohn RB, Brodsky JB, et al. Lateral thoracotomy and one-lung anesthesia in patients with morbid obesity. Ann Thorac Surg 1982;34(5):572–80.
62. Brodsky JB, Wyner J, Ehrenwerth J, et al. One-lung anesthesia in morbidly obese patients. Anesthesiology 1982;57(2):132–4.
63. Brodsky JB. Positioning the morbidly obese patient for anesthesia. Obes Surg 2002;12(6):751–8.
64. St Julien JB, Aldrich MC, Sheng S, et al. Obesity increases operating room time for lobectomy in the society of thoracic surgeons database. Ann Thorac Surg 2012;94(6):1841–7.
65. Kilic A, Schuchert MJ, Pennathur A, et al. Impact of obesity on perioperative outcomes of minimally invasive esophagectomy. Ann Thorac Surg 2009;87(2):412–5.
66. Okamura A, Watanabe M, Kurogochi T, et al. Mediastinal adiposity influences the technical difficulty of thoracic procedure in minimally invasive esophagectomy. World J Surg 2016;40(10):2398–404.
67. Banka G, Woodard G, Hernandez-Boussard T, et al. Laparoscopic vs open gastric bypass surgery: differences in patient demographics, safety, and outcomes. Arch Surg 2012;147(6):550–6.
68. Nguyen NT, Goldman C, Rosenquist CJ, et al. Laparoscopic versus open gastric bypass: a randomized study of outcomes, quality of life, and costs. Ann Surg 2001;234(3):279–89 [discussion: 289–91].
69. Lee J, Mabardy A, Kermani R, et al. Laparoscopic vs open ventral hernia repair in the era of obesity. JAMA Surg 2013;148(8):723–6.
70. Vargas GM, Sieloff EP, Parmar AD, et al. Laparoscopy decreases complications for obese patients undergoing elective rectal surgery. Surg Endosc 2016;30(5):1826–32.
71. Whitson BA, Andrade RS, Boettcher A, et al. Video-assisted thoracoscopic surgery is more favorable than thoracotomy for resection of clinical stage I non-small cell lung cancer. Ann Thorac Surg 2007;83(6):1965–70.
72. Villamizar NR, Darrabie MD, Burfeind WR, et al. Thoracoscopic lobectomy is associated with lower morbidity compared with thoracotomy. J Thorac Cardiovasc Surg 2009;138(2):419–25.
73. Flores RM, Park BJ, Dycoco J, et al. Lobectomy by video-assisted thoracic surgery (VATS) versus thoracotomy for lung cancer. J Thorac Cardiovasc Surg 2009;138(1):11–8.
74. Jeon JH, Kang CH, Kim HS, et al. Video-assisted thoracoscopic lobectomy in non-small-cell lung cancer patients with chronic obstructive pulmonary disease is associated with lower pulmonary complications than open lobectomy: a propensity score-matched analysis. Eur J Cardiothorac Surg 2014;45(4):640–5.
75. Ellsworth WA, Basu CB, Iverson RE. Perioperative considerations for patient safety during cosmetic surgery - preventing complications. Can J Plast Surg 2009;17(1):9–16.
76. Dybec RB. Intraoperative positioning and care of the obese patient. Plast Surg Nurs 2004;24(3):118–22.
77. Stein PD, Beemath A, Olson RE. Obesity as a risk factor in venous thromboembolism. Am J Med 2005;118(9):978–80.
78. Rocha AT, de Vasconcellos AG, da Luz Neto ER, et al. Risk of venous thromboembolism and efficacy of thromboprophylaxis in hospitalized obese medical patients and in obese patients undergoing bariatric surgery. Obes Surg 2006;16(12):1645–55.
79. Cooper L. Postoperative complications after thoracic surgery in the morbidly obese patient. Anesthesiol Res Pract 2011;2011:865634.
80. Chou R, Gordon DB, de Leon-Casasola OA, et al. Management of postoperative pain: a clinical practice guideline from the American Pain Society, the American Society of Regional Anesthesia and Pain Medicine, and the American Society of Anesthesiologists' Committee on Regional Anesthesia, Executive Committee, and Administrative Council. J Pain 2016;17(2):131–57.
81. Schumann R, Jones SB, Cooper B, et al. Update on best practice recommendations for anesthetic perioperative care and pain management in weight loss surgery, 2004-2007. Obesity (Silver Spring) 2009;17(5):889–94.
82. American Society of Anesthesiologists Task Force on Perioperative Management of Patients with Obstructive Sleep Apnea. Practice guidelines for the perioperative management of patients with obstructive sleep apnea: an updated report by the American Society of Anesthesiologists Task Force on Perioperative Management of Patients with Obstructive Sleep Apnea. Anesthesiology 2014;120(2):268–86.
83. von Ungern-Sternberg BS, Regli A, Reber A, et al. Effect of obesity and thoracic epidural analgesia on

perioperative spirometry. Br J Anaesth 2005;94(1): 121–7.
84. Kobayashi R, Mori S, Wakai K, et al. Paravertebral block via the surgical field versus epidural block for patients undergoing thoracotomy: a randomized clinical trial. Surg Today 2013;43(9):963–9.
85. Daly DJ, Myles PS. Update on the role of paravertebral blocks for thoracic surgery: are they worth it? Curr Opin Anaesthesiol 2009;22(1):38–43.
86. Davies RG, Myles PS, Graham JM. A comparison of the analgesic efficacy and side-effects of paravertebral vs epidural blockade for thoracotomy–a systematic review and meta-analysis of randomized trials. Br J Anaesth 2006;96(4):418–26.
87. Tamura T, Mori S, Mori A, et al. A randomized controlled trial comparing paravertebral block via the surgical field with thoracic epidural block using ropivacaine for post-thoracotomy pain relief. J Anesth 2017;31(2):263–70.
88. Simonsen DF, Søgaard M, Bozi I, et al. Risk factors for postoperative pneumonia after lung cancer surgery and impact of pneumonia on survival. Respir Med 2015;109(10):1340–6.
89. Agostini P, Cieslik H, Rathinam S, et al. Postoperative pulmonary complications following thoracic surgery: are there any modifiable risk factors? Thorax 2010;65(9):815–8.
90. Ploeg AJ, Kappetein AP, van Tongeren RB, et al. Factors associated with perioperative complications and long-term results after pulmonary resection for primary carcinoma of the lung. Eur J Cardiothorac Surg 2003;23(1):26–9.
91. Andalib A, Ramana-Kumar AV, Bartlett G, et al. Influence of postoperative infectious complications on long-term survival of lung cancer patients: a population-based cohort study. J Thorac Oncol 2013;8(5):554–61.
92. Atkins BZ, Shah AS, Hutcheson KA, et al. Reducing hospital morbidity and mortality following esophagectomy. Ann Thorac Surg 2004;78(4):1170–6 [discussion: 1170–6].
93. Eichenberger A, Proietti S, Wicky S, et al. Morbid obesity and postoperative pulmonary atelectasis: an underestimated problem. Anesth Analg 2002; 95(6):1788–92.
94. Launer H, Nguyen DV, Cooke DT. National perioperative outcomes of pulmonary lobectomy for cancer in the obese patient: a propensity score matched analysis. J Thorac Cardiovasc Surg 2013;145(5):1312–8.
95. Miao L, Chen H, Xiang J, et al. A high body mass index in esophageal cancer patients is not associated with adverse outcomes following esophagectomy. J Cancer Res Clin Oncol 2015;141(5): 941–50.
96. Mungo B, Zogg CK, Hooker CM, et al. Does obesity affect the outcomes of pulmonary resections for lung cancer? A National Surgical Quality Improvement Program analysis. Surgery 2015;157(4):792–800.
97. Ferguson MK, Im HK, Watson S, et al. Association of body mass index and outcomes after major lung resection. Eur J Cardiothorac Surg 2014;45(4): e94–9 [discussion: e99].
98. Kozower BD, Sheng S, O'Brien SM, et al. STS database risk models: predictors of mortality and major morbidity for lung cancer resection. Ann Thorac Surg 2010;90(3):875–81 [discussion: 881–3].
99. Smith PW, Wang H, Gazoni LM, et al. Obesity does not increase complications after anatomic resection for non-small cell lung cancer. Ann Thorac Surg 2007;84(4):1098–105 [discussion: 1105–6].
100. Bhayani NH, Gupta A, Dunst CM, et al. Does morbid obesity worsen outcomes after esophagectomy? Ann Thorac Surg 2013;95(5):1756–61.
101. Gould MK, Garcia DA, Wren SM, et al. Prevention of VTE in nonorthopedic surgical patients: antithrombotic therapy and prevention of thrombosis, 9th ed: American College of Chest Physicians Evidence-Based Clinical Practice Guidelines. Chest 2012;141(2 Suppl):e227S–277.
102. Stein PD, Matta F. Pulmonary embolism and deep venous thrombosis following bariatric surgery. Obes Surg 2013;23(5):663–8.
103. Tjeertes EK, Hoeks SE, Beks SB, et al. Obesity–a risk factor for postoperative complications in general surgery? BMC Anesthesiol 2015;15:112.
104. Olsen MA, Lock-Buckley P, Hopkins D, et al. The risk factors for deep and superficial chest surgical-site infections after coronary artery bypass graft surgery are different. J Thorac Cardiovasc Surg 2002;124(1):136–45.
105. Lilienfeld DE, Vlahov D, Tenney JH, et al. Obesity and diabetes as risk factors for postoperative wound infections after cardiac surgery. Am J Infect Control 1988;16(1):3–6.
106. Grauhan O, Navasardyan A, Hofmann M, et al. Prevention of poststernotomy wound infections in obese patients by negative pressure wound therapy. J Thorac Cardiovasc Surg 2013;145(5): 1387–92.
107. Melis M, Meredith KL, Weber J, et al. Body mass index and perioperative complications after esophagectomy for cancer. Ann Surg 2015. [Epub ahead of print].
108. Melis M, Weber J, Shridhar R, et al. Body mass index and perioperative complications after oesophagectomy for adenocarcinoma: a systematic database review. BMJ Open 2013;3(5) [pii: e001336].
109. Thomas PA, Berbis J, Falcoz PE, et al. National perioperative outcomes of pulmonary lobectomy for cancer: the influence of nutritional status.

Eur J Cardiothorac Surg 2014;45(4):652–9 [discussion: 659].

110. Konda P, Ai D, Guerra CE, et al. Identification of risk factors associated with postoperative acute kidney injury after esophagectomy for esophageal cancer. J Cardiothorac Vasc Anesth 2017;31(2):474–81.
111. Blom RL, Lagarde SM, Klinkenbijl JH, et al. A high body mass index in esophageal cancer patients does not influence postoperative outcome or long-term survival. Ann Surg Oncol 2012;19(3): 766–71.
112. Healy LA, Ryan AM, Gopinath B, et al. Impact of obesity on outcomes in the management of localized adenocarcinoma of the esophagus and esophagogastric junction. J Thorac Cardiovasc Surg 2007;134(5):1284–91.
113. Kayani B, Okabayashi K, Ashrafian H, et al. Does obesity affect outcomes in patients undergoing esophagectomy for cancer? A meta-analysis. World J Surg 2012;36(8):1785–95.
114. Attaran S, McShane J, Whittle I, et al. A propensity-matched comparison of survival after lung resection in patients with a high versus low body mass index. Eur J Cardiothorac Surg 2012;42(4):653–8.
115. Williams T, Gulack BC, Kim S, et al. Operative risk for major lung resection increases at extremes of body mass index. Ann Thorac Surg 2017;103(1): 296–302.
116. Mullen JT, Moorman DW, Davenport DL. The obesity paradox: body mass index and outcomes in patients undergoing nonbariatric general surgery. Ann Surg 2009;250(1):166–72.

Thoracic Surgery Considerations in the Child and Young Adult

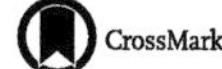

Marvin D. Atkins, MD[a], Stephanie Fuller, MD, MS[b,*]

KEYWORDS

• Vascular ring • Pulmonary artery sling • Tracheobronchial compression • Congenital heart surgery

KEY POINTS

- Various pathologic aortic arch anomalies or cardiomegaly from congenital heart disease can lead to significant compression of the trachea, bronchii, and/or the esophagus.
- As a general rule, neonates and infants present with airway issues, whereas dysphagia tends to occur more widely in older children and adults.
- A vascular ring may be suggested on chest radiography by the nonspecific findings of a pulmonary infiltrate, atelectasis, unilateral or bilateral hyperinflation, or the aortic arch position.
- Barium esophagogram has been replaced by computed tomography angiography and cardiac gated MRI in the assessment of aortic arch anomalies.
- Vascular rings or slings may result in important obstructive airway or esophageal symptoms, necessitating division of the ring or relocation of the sling.

INTRODUCTION

Thoracic surgery in the pediatric population encompasses a vast array of pathologies, including problems of the trachea and airway, esophagus, diaphragm, lungs, chest wall, heart, and great vessels. Many of these conditions are managed by the general pediatric surgeon and represent a core component of that specialty. For example, disorders such as esophageal atresia, tracheoesophageal fistula, congenital diaphragmatic hernia, chest wall deformities, and bronchopulmonary malformations (congenital pulmonary airway malformation, pulmonary sequestration, congenital lobar emphysema and bronchogenic cyst) fall under the purview of the general pediatric surgeon. As such, these disorders are not covered in this issue of *Thoracic Surgery Clinics*.

The congenital heart surgeon manages all disorders in the pediatric population involving the heart, great vessels, and central airway, including compression of the trachea/bronchii and esophagus from vascular structures or their remnants and congenital tracheal stenosis. Vascular pathology involving the trachea and bronchi are typically managed in conjunction with either the pediatric surgeon or the pediatric otolaryngologist. Because many of these neonates and children with primary tracheal and bronchial pathology also have associated congenital heart defects, most often as a part of a syndromic disorder (such as VACTERL [vertebral, anal, cardiac, tracheoesophageal, renal, limb defects]), a congenital heart surgeon is typically involved in their care.

Disclosure Statement: Neither author has any financial or commercial interest or disclosures relevant to the content of this article.

[a] Cardiothoracic Surgery, Division of Cardiothoracic Surgery, The Hospital of the University of Pennsylvania, 3400 Civic Center Boulevard, Philadelphia, PA 19014, USA; [b] Division of Cardiothoracic Surgery, The Perelman School of Medicine, University of Pennsylvania, The Children's Hospital of Philadelphia, 3401 Civic Center Boulevard, Suite 12NW10, Philadelphia, PA 19014, USA
* Corresponding author.
E-mail address: fullers@email.chop.edu

Thorac Surg Clin 28 (2018) 43–52
https://doi.org/10.1016/j.thorsurg.2017.08.005

This article reviews commonly encountered pathologic vascular anomalies associated with tracheobronchial disorders as well as primary tracheal disorders that are encountered in a pediatric cardiothoracic practice.

EMBRYOLOGY

By 5 weeks of fetal development, the primordial heart tubes have fused and 6 paired aortic arches form connecting the dorsal and ventral aortae. The arches develop serially. That is, the first and second arches followed by the third and fourth, then the fifth and sixth. In normal development, the first and second arches undergo near complete involution with minor contributions to the facial arteries. Septation of the conotruncus forms the proximal ascending aorta and the proximal pulmonary artery. The distal ascending aorta, the aortic arch until the left common carotid artery, and the innominate artery derive from the aortic sac. The third aortic arch forms the bilateral carotid arteries. The left fourth aortic arch forms the distal aortic arch, aortic isthmus, and joins the truncus arteriosus contributing to the ascending aorta. Normally a portion of the right fourth aortic arch involutes, leaving the standard leftward aortic arch. The remaining components of the right fourth arch contributes to the development of the right subclavian artery. The ventral portion of the sixth arch interacts with the lung bud to form the remaining pulmonary artery. The dorsal right sixth aortic arch involutes, whereas the dorsal left sixth aortic arch forms the ductus arteriosus. The left subclavian artery forms from the left intersegmental artery. The descending thoracic aorta is formed from the left dorsal aorta (**Fig. 1**).

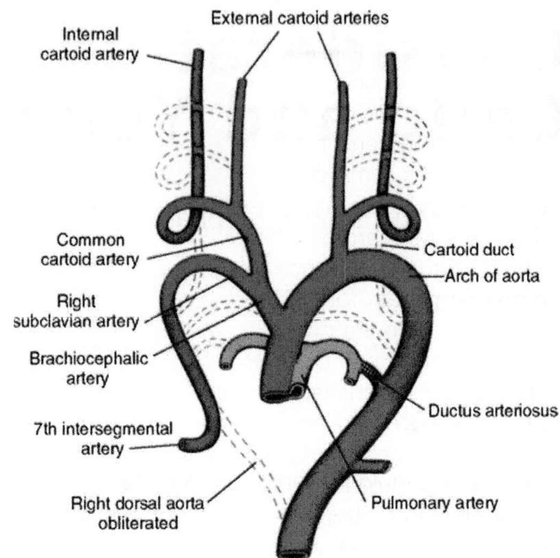

Fig. 1. Normal left aortic arch development from the 6 paired aortic arches that connect the dorsal and ventral aortae. The opaque arches represent normal programmed cell death and involution.

This complex interaction between the involution or programmed cell death, and migration or persistence of the various portions of the aortic arches and dorsal or ventral aortae results in variant anatomy. The outcome can range from an inconsequential variant to life threatening with partial or complete vascular rings causing severe tracheal compression. Aortic arch anomalies producing tracheoesophageal constriction account for 1% to 2% of all congenital heart defects.

Diagnosis

Significant airway compression may occur owing to such pathologic vascular anomalies or even from underlying congenital heart disease and cardiomegaly itself. Airway compression is often unrecognized on prenatal ultrasound imaging. Neonates can present with dyspnea, wheezing, and stridor that may be life threatening. There may also be symptoms of feeding difficulties and dysphagia with cardiovascular-related compression. As a general rule, neonates present with airway issues, whereas dysphagia tends to occur more widely in older children and adults.

Evaluation of the neonate or child with suspected tracheobronchial compression may include anteroposterior and lateral chest radiographs, barium esophagram, echocardiogram, computed tomography (CT) angiography (CTA) or cardiac MRI, and direct microlaryngoscopy and bronchoscopy. When fine resolution of the airway is not necessary, cardiac MRI is preferred to CTA as because it avoids ionizing radiation in children.[1,2] A disadvantage of MRI is the significant time needed for image acquisition and the necessity to provide sedation, especially in the neonate and infant. A normal frontal and lateral chest radiograph may increase the likelihood of finding a vascular ring, because the vast majority of vascular rings are associated with a right aortic arch.[3] Microlaryngoscopy and bronchoscopy can also help to identify synchronous primary airway lesions that may be present, as well as help document vocal cord motion before cardiovascular surgery. Often it is helpful in distinguishing tracheomalacia from true compression.

By far, the majority of vascular rings are associated with a right-sided aortic arch. The most prevalent vascular anomalies that result in airway or esophageal compression are (in decreasing order of frequency): (1) double aortic arch, (2) right aortic arch with aberrant left subclavian artery originating from a retroesophageal diverticulum (diverticulum of Kommerell), (3) innominate artery compression,

(4) left aortic arch with aberrant right subclavian artery, and (5) pulmonary artery sling.[3] Left aortic arch with aberrant right subclavian artery, emanating as the most distal aortic arch structure, is highly prevalent in the general population but rarely causes symptoms. This is often considered a normal variant in the context of asymptomatic individuals. Furthermore, although right aortic arch with mirror image branching pattern is considered a normal variant for right arches, a vascular ring may form from the presence of a left ligamentum arteriosum to complete the ring. This circumstance can be challenging to diagnose because there is no obvious retroesophageal diverticulum, but rather the only evidence of the ring may be a small leftward-directed dimple off the aorta. We consider these vascular anomalies in further detail.

Complete vascular rings

Complete vascular rings include double aortic arch and right aortic arch with aberrant left subclavian artery originating from a retroesophageal diverticulum and associated left ligamentum arteriosum (**Fig. 2**).

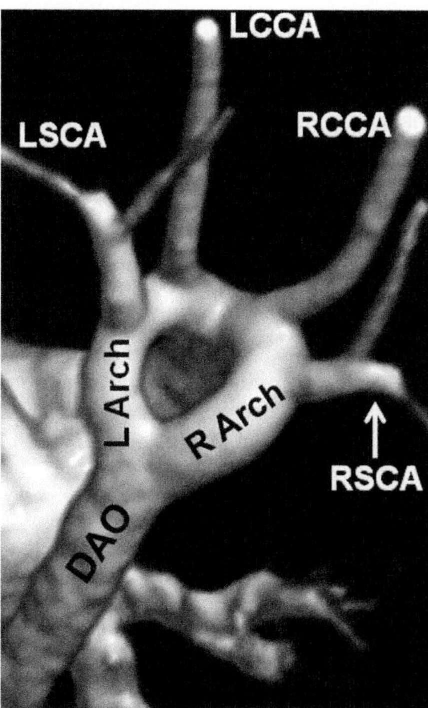

Fig. 2. Magnetic resonance angiogram of an unobstructed double aortic arch viewed from right posterior oblique with cranial angulation. Note that the right aortic arch is slightly larger. DAO, descending aorta; L Arch, left-sided arch; LCCA, left common carotid artery; LSCA, left subclavian artery; R Arch, right-sided arch; RCCA, right common carotid artery; RSCA, right subclavian artery. (*Courtesy of* Matthew Harris, MD, Philadelphia, PA.)

With true vascular rings, the trachea and esophagus are anatomically completely surrounded and compressed. Sometimes the mainstem bronchi may be narrowed. Symptoms involve biphasic stridor, wheezing, cyanosis with feeding, recurrent pneumonias or lower airway infections, and dysphagia. Dysphagia owing to external compression of the esophagus from a vascular structure is termed dysphagia lusoria. Patients may describe food hanging up in the mid to upper esophagus and have associated weight loss.

Initial diagnostic testing includes barium esophagram and airway fluoroscopy. This testing often shows a posterior indentation of the esophagus on lateral views. Cardiac MR angiography will define the vascular and tracheal anatomy. Esophagoscopy reveals pulsatility at the site of obstruction, as does bronchoscopy. Double aortic arches account for 50% to 60% of vascular rings and are the most frequent cause of vascular compression of the airway in children.[4,5] Because they are complete and tight, they are often symptomatic early in infancy and most often require surgical correction by dividing the smaller, nondominant arch. Because the right aortic arch is typically dominant, the left aortic arch via the left chest is divided at the time of surgical management. Approximately 30% of patients undergoing surgical correction will still exhibit symptoms after surgery owing to weakness of the cartilaginous rings from longstanding compression.[5] If severe symptoms do not resolve over time as the cartilage matures and stiffens, then a tracheostomy may need to be placed.

A right aortic arch with left ligamentum arteriosum and aberrant left subclavian artery also encircles both the trachea and esophagus. This configuration is not usually as constricting and thus often is asymptomatic or presents with symptoms later in life, sometimes when solids are introduced. This entity is the second most frequently occurring vascular ring and accounts for 12% to 25% of cases.[4] Surgical correction involves division of the left ligamentum arteriosum. Most also proceed with either aortopexy or resection of the diverticulum. Kommerell's diverticulum is the outpouching of the descending aorta that embryologically derives from ductus arteriosus tissue. The fibrous left ligamentum segment is in continuity with the diverticulum (but not observed on MRI or CT angiograms) and therefore completes the ring as it is tethered inferiorly to the left pulmonary artery. The left subclavian artery originates at the retroesophageal diverticulum. If the ring were divided and the retroesophageal diverticulum left intact, this can result in late compression of the trachea or esophagus.[5]

Innominate artery compression

The innominate artery can cause tracheal compression if it originates more distal than usual on the aortic arch and then must cross anterior to the trachea toward the right. This may manifest as a focal anterior tracheal compression at the level just proximal to the carina. Bronchoscopy exhibits focal, pulsatile, and asymmetric airway compression just proximal to the carina and of the right mainstem bronchus. Definitive diagnosis can be made with MRI or CTA examination. Deformity of the tracheal rings and resultant cartilaginous weakness may compound the problem and result in persistent airway symptoms despite surgical intervention. In mildly affected patients, conservative monitoring is all that is needed; patients can improve as the airway grows and the cartilaginous rings become more rigid. However, with severely affected children, surgical correction in the form of aortopexy with suspension of the innominate artery to the undersurface of the sternum may be needed. Reimplantation or transection of the innominate artery may be another surgical option.[6,7]

Pulmonary artery sling

Pulmonary artery sling involves an anomalous course of the left pulmonary artery, which originates from the posterior aspect of the right pulmonary artery instead of from the common pulmonary artery trunk (**Fig. 3**). In contrast with vascular rings, where the ring includes the trachea and the esophagus, in pulmonary sling the anomalous left pulmonary artery passes in between the trachea and esophagus as it courses toward the left hilum, compressing the distal trachea and right mainstem bronchus as well as the anterior aspect of the esophagus. Although a rare entity, pulmonary artery slings are often associated with other severe abnormalities. Approximately 50% have congenital heart disease (most commonly tetralogy of Fallot), 50% have other congenital anomalies, 50% have complete cartilaginous tracheal rings, and others have tracheomalacia, abnormal pulmonary lobulations, or bronchus suis (right upper lobe bronchus originating directly from the trachea).[4] Importantly, the workup of these children should not only include CTA or cardiac MRI/MR angiography imaging, it should also include a bronchoscopy to evaluate the airway before cardiac surgery. Repairing the tracheal stenosis and the pulmonary artery sling at the same time is associated with better prognosis.[5] Mild cases can be monitored; however, if significant respiratory symptoms are present, then surgical translocation and reimplantation of the left pulmonary artery may be needed. If the tracheal stenosis is limited, a tracheal resection can be done at the same must be performed with the repair of the pulmonary artery sling.

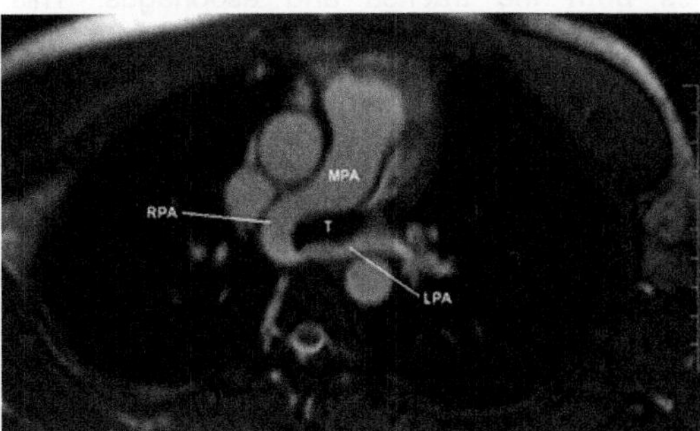

Fig. 3. Axial cut of an magnetic resonance angiogram showing a pulmonary artery sling. In this disease, the left pulmonary artery originates from the proximal right pulmonary artery and then passes between the relatively anterior trachea and the relatively posterior esophagus as it heads back toward the left lung. This creates a sling around the trachea with a leftward pull typically producing severe tracheal symptoms. MPA, main pulmonary artery; LPA, left pulmonary artery; RPA, right pulmonary artery.

Other vascular abnormalities

An aberrant right subclavian artery, as the last branch emanating from the left-sided aortic arch, may result in posterior compression of the esophagus as the aberrant right subclavian artery courses behind the esophagus. Dysphagia can be a presenting symptom, but most often this entity is asymptomatic.[3] A cervical aortic arch is a rare entity and occurs when the aortic arch abnormally courses high into the neck superior to the clavicles (potentially as high as C2). Although typically people with isolated cervical aortic arch are asymptomatic, symptoms of pulsatile cervical mass, respiratory symptoms, and/or dysphagia may be present and ultimately depend on the variant present.

CONGENITAL CARDIAC MALFORMATIONS

Acyanotic or cyanotic congenital heart disease can result in direct compression of the airways or lungs with resultant respiratory symptoms and represents an underappreciated cause of such symptoms. The trachea, carina, and left mainstem bronchus are closely associated with various cardiac structures, such as the left atrium, left pulmonary artery, and left pulmonary veins. It, therefore, seems that various cardiac pathologies resulting in dilation/enlargement of cardiac structures or massive cardiomegaly may lead to airway compression and symptoms. Congenital heart disease resulting in left-to-right shunting (such as with ventricular septal defects, patent ductus arteriosus, or atrioventricular canal), tetralogy of Fallot with absent pulmonary valve leaflets syndrome or pulmonary atresia, mitral regurgitation, truncus arteriosus, or dilated cardiomyopathy may be sources of airway compression. Increased intracardiac filling pressures may lead to enlarged bronchial vessels and lymphatics, and thus ultimately to intraluminal bronchial edema and obstruction.[4] In addition to cardiac MRI, echocardiography, and bronchoscopy, some patients may benefit from cardiac catheterization to delineate cardiac pathology and potential effects on the airway. If possible, the underlying cardiac defect should be addressed to improve the airway issues. Furthermore, patients with complex structural heart disease who undergo interventional catheterization for balloon dilation and stent implantation of a branch pulmonary artery may experience ipsilateral mainstem bronchus compression.[8]

PRIMARY DISORDERS OF THE TRACHEA AND BRONCHUS

Congenital tracheal and bronchial anomalies can present acutely within the first few days of life with potentially fatal respiratory distress or remain asymptomatic and undiagnosed for many years. Immediate diagnosis and appropriate intervention can allow tracheal growth and prevent morbidity and mortality. Neonates may present in respiratory distress or alternatively with the symptom of noisy breathing, particularly on exertion. Stridor is most often due to laryngomalacia. However, a normal laryngoscopic examination should warrant further investigation of potential tracheal or bronchial anomalies. Delineation of the lower airways and cardiovascular anatomy with microlaryngoscopy and bronchoscopy and radiologic imaging (CTA; or MR angiography) is critical for accurate diagnosis and development of a management plan. Ultimately, congenital anomalies of the trachea and bronchi result from either an intrinsic abnormality of the cartilage or extrinsic compression of the airway from cardiovascular or gastrointestinal malformations. A multidisciplinary approach with the collaboration of anesthesiologists, cardiologists, cardiothoracic surgeons, general pediatric surgeons, neonatal and pediatric intensivists, and pediatric otolaryngologists specializing in airway reconstruction is necessary for effective management of congenital airway disease. Tracheomalacia (both primary and secondary), congenital cardiovascular abnormalities, tracheoesophageal fistula with esophageal atresia, tracheal stenosis, and foregut duplication cysts can all lead to airway compromise.

Tracheomalacia is the most prevalent pathology affecting the trachea for both full-term and premature neonates. Tracheomalacia is a dynamic narrowing of the lumen of the trachea during breathing owing to a weakness of the trachea wall. The trachea is composed of 16 to 20 C-shaped cartilaginous rings anteriorly and a soft membranous trachealis muscle posteriorly. The tracheal lumen normally undergoes dynamic changes during the respiratory cycle; however, the degree of airway collapse is excessive in patients with tracheomalacia and results in symptoms.[9] Most instances of tracheomalacia are intrathoracic, with tracheal narrowing seen with forced expiration or cough. Extrathoracic tracheomalacia occurs during inspiration when negative intrapleural pressures are transmitted to the extrathoracic trachea.[10] Pathologic tracheomalacia is typically seen when the tracheal lumen narrows by more than 50%. The normal tracheal ratio of the cartilaginous ring to the posterior membranous wall ranges from 4:1 to 5:1 and changes to between 2:1 and 3:1 with pathologic tracheomalacia resulting in the development of symptoms. Symptoms of tracheomalacia may include cough (83%), recurrent lower airways infection (63%), dyspnea (59%), recurrent wheeze (49%), recurrent rattling (48%), reduced exercise tolerance (35%), symptoms of reflux (26%), retractions (19%), and stridor (28%).[11] These findings are often more prevalent with increased activity or agitation. Patients with tracheomalacia may also present with recurrent respiratory infections owing to impaired clearance of secretions with luminal collapse. Patients with intrathoracic tracheomalacia present with a wheeze on expiration, whereas patients with extrathoracic tracheomalacia present with stridor on inspiration.[9] Infants with extrinsic vascular compression may also present with feeding difficulties such as dysphagia, regurgitation, and coughing and cyanosis with feeding.

History and physical examination findings can be combined with results from pulmonary function tests and radiologic imaging studies to narrow the differential diagnoses and determine the etiology. Pulmonary function testing may show a truncated expiratory flow/volume loop in older children, but are not as helpful in infants owing to the need for sedation. Fluoroscopy can be used to look for an anteroposterior luminal decrease in diameter with a specificity of 96% to 100%. However, this modality is poorly sensitive (23%–62%) for tracheomalacia because, during periods of crying, the anteroposterior diameter can decrease by up to 50% in a normal infant trachea.[9] Barium esophagography can be used to discern a tracheoesophageal fistula or vascular ring. CT and MRI performed with contrast can help to evaluate external compression of the trachea, when looking for either masses or vascular compression. MRI/MR angiography is considered preferable to CT because it does not involve radiation exposure; however, CT may be the ideal study in a more medically fragile patient because it can be performed much quicker and is more sensitive for the airway. Modern CT imaging can help to image the airway during the different phases of respiration, thus making it easier to detect dynamic changes in caliber. However, there are a few concerns with this method. First, it requires radiation exposure. Moreover, in infants, this requires the patient to be sedated and intubated, which can distort the airway and change the tracheal dynamics.[9] The best way to evaluate for tracheomalacia remains flexible bronchoscopy under spontaneous ventilation. Dynamic movements of the airway during inspiration can be masked with heavy sedation, use of a paralytic agent, or with positive pressure ventilation, resulting in a false-negative result. Currently the challenge remains that the diagnosis of tracheomalacia is largely subjective, determined by the bronchoscopist because there is no standard definition at this time. Tracheomalacia may be associated with many conditions. Cardiovascular anomalies are associated in up to 50% of patients with tracheomalacia. These anomalies include septal defects of the atrium or ventricle, patent ductus arteriosus, tetralogy of Fallot, abnormalities of the aortic arch, hypoplastic left or right heart, dextrocardia, and valvular stenosis. Bronchopulmonary dysplasia is seen in up to 52% of infants with tracheomalacia. Gastroesophageal reflux has been seen in up to 78% of patients with tracheomalacia that is severe or life threatening. Secondary airway lesions, including subglottic stenosis, laryngomalacia, and vocal cord paralysis, are also seen in patients with tracheomalacia. There is also thought to be a neurologic relationship, because one-half of patients with tracheomalacia have an associated neurologic impairment and one-quarter of patients have a severe developmental delay.

Primary Tracheomalacia

Congenital or primary tracheomalacia results from inadequate maturity of the tracheal cartilage itself owing either to premature birth, or to an inherent immaturity or abnormality of the cartilage matrix itself. Congenital tracheomalacia may occur in full-term infants, but more usually is seen in premature infants. The overall incidence of primary tracheomalacia has been reported to be 1 in 2100 children by conservative estimates.[11] Primary tracheomalacia has been associated with numerous conditions including Ehlers-Danlos syndrome, mucopolysaccharidosis, CHARGE (coloboma of the eye, heart defects, choanal atresia, retardation of growth, ear abnormalities and deafness), VACTERL/VATER anomaly (vertebral anomalies, anal atresia, cardiac defects, tracheoesophageal fistula and/or esophageal atresia, renal and radial anomalies and limb defects), trisomy 21, Pfeiffer syndrome, DiGeorge syndrome, Pierre Robin sequence, and tracheoesophageal fistula. Some may consider tracheomalacia associated with tracheoesophageal fistula as a secondary form, but many feel it is really a primary form of tracheomalacia, because the weakness of the trachea is not caused by external compression, but rather is due to an inherent weakness of the involved tracheal cartilage. Most patients do not require any intervention and improve over time with maturation of the infant and airway; most resolve by 2 years of age.[11] In rare instances, a tracheotomy and positive-pressure ventilation may be needed for infants with growth derangements, persistent respiratory distress, or feeding difficulties. Some have used endotracheal or endobronchial stents. However, owing to the inherent small nature of the pediatric airway, these should not be used to avoid problems with extrusion, migration, bleeding, granulation tissue, difficulty with removal, pneumonia, and death. Endotracheal or endobronchial stents should be reserved for emergent situations and require close surveillance of the airway. More recently, 3-dimensional printed, bioresorbable splints have been described and surgically placed for life-threatening tracheobronchomalacia in children.[12]

Acquired or Secondary Tracheomalacia

Acquired or secondary tracheomalacia is due to compression on the airway, which may be from a variety of sources including cardiovascular (as discussed elsewhere in this article), gastrointestinal, musculoskeletal, or neoplastic etiologies. This compression results in both a direct narrowing of the lumen as well as a weakening of the tracheal cartilage. A frequently occurring etiology is prolonged endotracheal intubation and associated insults of increased airway pressure, oxygen toxicity, and recurrent infections.[10] In premature infants with respiratory distress syndrome, this is compounded by an inherent immaturity of the tracheal cartilage itself. Another cause is tracheostomy placement. The surgical appliance may weaken the suprastomal trachea and the trachea adjacent to a cuff on the tracheostomy tube. Additionally, compression may be due to a cervical or thoracic tumor, cyst, or abscess. Skeletal pathology, such as thoracic dysplasia, may also result in secondary tracheomalacia. The treatment of secondary tracheomalacia relies on alleviating the underlying cause of the external compression. It is notable that, even after addressing the underlying compressive etiology, the tracheomalacia may continue owing to the weakening and dysmorphia of the cartilage.

TRACHEAL WEBS

Membranous tracheal webs are rare and considerably less frequent than airway narrowing from cartilaginous defects or laryngeal webs.[13] They occur at the level of the cricoid and are usually treated by endoscopic means. These webs can be incised sharply with an instrument or with a laser followed by balloon dilation. More extensive webs may need treatment with tracheal resection.

CONGENITAL TRACHEAL STENOSIS

Congenital tracheal stenosis (CTS) involves at least 50% narrowing of the tracheal lumen and may encompass a few rings or even the entire trachea. If the tracheal rings grow out of proportion to the posterior membranous trachea, complete or near complete tracheal rings may be formed. In contrast with the normal "C-shaped" rings of a normal trachea, complete tracheal rings are narrower and are believed to be restricted in growth. Most children with CTS and complete tracheal rings present during infancy. Symptoms include biphasic stridor, expiratory stridor, retractions, cyanosis, apnea, chest congestion, and respiratory distress. Patients may also be identified at time of a difficult intubation or subsequently from difficult intubations, which result in airway edema and granulation tissue that can acutely worsen an already narrow and marginalized airway. Patients may not become symptomatic until after a few months of age, as infants' respiratory needs "outgrow" their restricted airway. Moreover, a respiratory illness might unmask CTS, because symptoms sometimes progress rapidly. CTS and complete tracheal rings are usually associated with cardiovascular anomalies and thus require a full evaluation with preoperative imaging with CTA or cardiac MRI/MR angiography. In 1 large series, 71% of patients presented with cardiovascular anomalies; left pulmonary artery sling was the most frequent entity (48%). It is important to identify these cardiovascular anomalies because they can be corrected contemporaneously with tracheal repair.[14] Besides associated cardiovascular anomalies, infants with CTS may have pulmonary anomalies, Down syndrome, and Pfeiffer syndrome. Initial management is centered on providing respiratory support. This is often a challenging situation as even the smallest (2.0) endotracheal tube may not bypass the stenosis. Thus, often a "high" nasotracheal intubation is necessary with the endotracheal tube just through the vocal cords. This has to be carefully positioned such that the end of the endotracheal tube does not rub against the proximal, narrowed complete tracheal ring, which may lead to progressive mucosal edema and inflammation or granulation tissue, both leading to potential inability to ventilate. To avoid this situation, efforts should be made to support the airway without intubation. In situations where the infant cannot be safely and effectively ventilated even with intubation, extracorporeal membranous oxygenation may be performed to bridge to a definitive reconstructive surgery. Before tracheal reconstructive surgery, bronchoscopy is essential in delineating the tracheal stenosis, measuring the degree of narrowing, and the length of the narrowing. For situations where a severe stenosis precludes the passage of a bronchoscope for full airway visualization, CT imaging of the airway with fine cuts can render a full picture of the airway. A larger caliber airway in a patient who is overall stable may be monitored. However, most patients with CTS will need surgical correction.

In the past, CTS has been repaired with tracheal resection and anastomosis, cartilage graft augmentation, and patch tracheoplasty with a material such as pericardium. However, the gold standard has become the use of slide tracheoplasty (**Figs. 4** and **5**). Surgeons do have the option of performing a tracheal resection and anastomosis if only a few rings are involved. This should only be considered an option if there are no more than four or five rings involved. In performing a tracheal resection, 25% to 30% of the trachea can be removed before excessive anastomotic tension and threat of tracheal dehiscence precludes this as a therapeutic option.[15] However, even such a short span is often now managed with slide tracheoplasty. Slide tracheoplasty offers several advantages over previously described techniques including use of autologous tracheal tissue, earlier extubation, avoidance of a stent, decreased granulation tissue formation, and distribution of tension over a longer anastomotic length. Slide tracheoplasty shortens the trachea by half of the involved stenotic segment instead of the full length as would be required with a traditional tracheal resection approach. A slide tracheoplasty

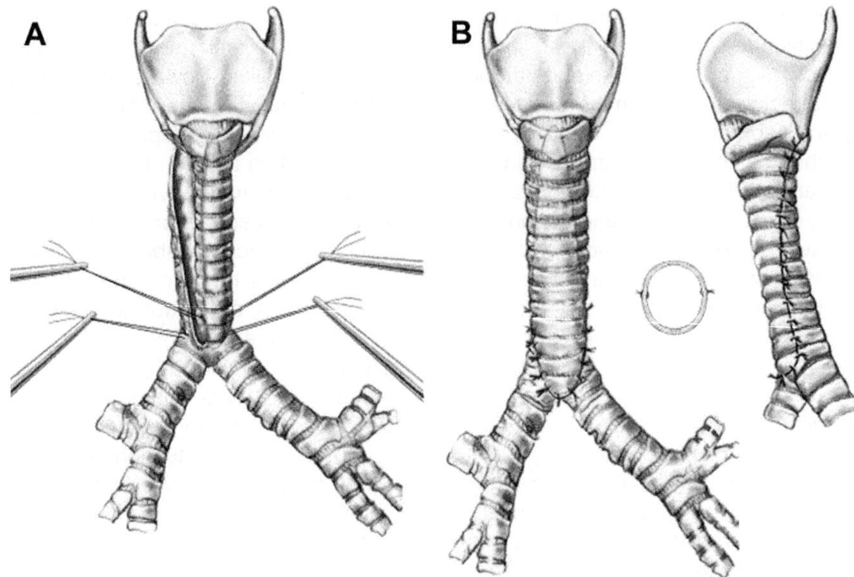

Fig. 4. Slide tracheoplasty. The trachea is divided transversely at the midpoint of the stenotic section. The trachea is freed up from its deep attachments to help increase segment mobility. Next, an anterior longitudinal incision is made in the proximal segment through the stenotic area until normal tracheal cartilage is encountered. (*A*) A posterior, longitudinal incision is made in the distal segment through the stenotic area until normal trachea or carina is encountered. The corners are trimmed and the tracheal segments are then slid over each other. (*B*) A running polydioxanone or Prolene suture is used to perform the anastomosis. (*From* Le Bret E, Garabédian EN, Teissier N, et al. Slide cricotracheoplasty in an infant. J Thorac Cardiovasc Surg 2006;132:180; with permission.)

may be performed from cricoid to carina if required. Briefly, the trachea is divided at the midpoint of the stenotic section, the trachea is freed up from its deep attachments down to the level of the carina and superiorly toward the larynx to help increase segment mobility. Lateral tracheal attachments are preserved to help decrease any potential damage to the tracheal vascular supply.

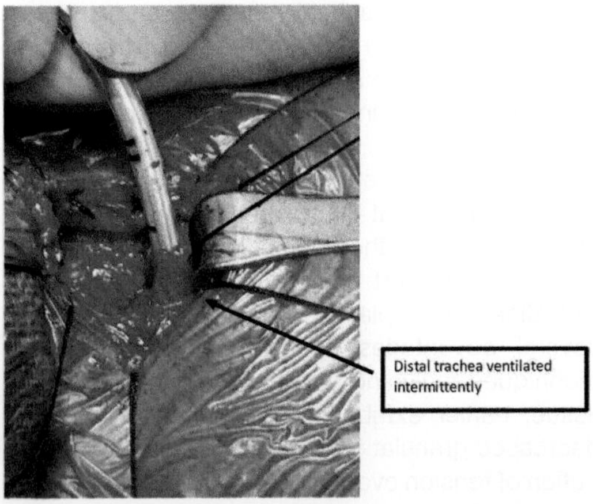

Fig. 5. Cervical tracheal exposure for slide tracheoplasty: using intermittent jet ventilation in the distal trachea, the trachea is prepared as in **Fig. 4** for slide tracheoplasty.

Next, an anterior longitudinal incision is made in the proximal segment through the stenotic area until normal tracheal cartilage is encountered. A posterior, longitudinal incision is made in the distal segment through the stenotic area until normal trachea or carina is encountered. The corners are trimmed and the tracheal segments are then slid over each other. A running polydioxanone or Prolene suture is used to perform the anastomosis. The slide can be extended into the anterior aspect of the cricoid or even into a bronchus if needed. Potential complications include recurrent laryngeal nerve injury, dehiscence and restenosis, and dysphagia. Postoperatively, bronchoscopy is performed to monitor and help mold the healing process through adjuvant techniques such as excision of granulation tissue and balloon dilation.

TRACHEAL CARTILAGINOUS SLEEVE

Tracheal cartilaginous sleeve (complete tracheal rings) is a rare tracheal anomaly in which the trachea forms as a long cylindrical sleeve of cartilage rather than with normal tracheal rings. The posterior membranous trachea is absent or greatly diminished. The sleeve may be restricted to the trachea alone or may extend into the bronchial tree. Respiratory distress results from restricted growth of the caliber and length of the airway, and from mucous plugging. Tracheal cartilaginous sleeve is mostly seen in craniosynostosis syndromes such as Apert, Crouzon, and Pfeiffer syndromes. The prognosis is poor with 1 report finding 90% of patients with both tracheal sleeves and craniosynostosis syndromes were dead by 2 years of age with 58% of the mortalities owing to airway pathology. In that series, the mean age of death is younger than 3 years in essentially all patients with complete tracheal rings.[16] The poor compliance of the cartilaginous sleeve is thought to result in issues with granulation tissue, functional issues, poor airway clearance mechanisms, and mucous plugging, which can be life threatening.[17] Tracheostomy is often necessary to bypass upper airway pathology and allow for pulmonary clearance of the airway. However, owing to the rigidity and abnormal configuration of the airway, tracheotomy in this population may be challenging and fraught with issues with granulation tissue and plugging, requiring frequent monitoring for this. Symptoms include respiratory distress, cyanosis, recurrent respiratory infections and croup, severe biphasic stridor, and failure to thrive. Bronchoscopic visualization is necessary for diagnosis and elucidation of the extent of the sleeve. Fine-cut CT imaging of the airway can also help to visualize tracheal configuration. Treatment options include tracheostomy for airway support, tracheal resection for short segments, or slide tracheoplasty for longer segments.

AGENESIS AND ATRESIA OF THE TRACHEA

This rare tracheal anomaly involves the complete or partial absence of the trachea and is sometimes seen with a tracheoesophageal fistula. The incidence is 1 in 50,000 live births with a 2:1 male predominance. Reportedly, 52% of affected individuals are premature, 50% to 94% are associated with other congenital malformations, and at least 50% involve pregnancies with polyhydramnios.[18] The Floyd classification is the most widely used system for tracheal agenesis. Type I (13%) has an absent proximal trachea with distal tracheoesophageal fistula. Type II (65%) has a complete absence of the trachea with the carina usually opening into the esophagus, but not always. Type III (22%) has the origin of both mainstem bronchi directly from the esophagus.[19] Immediately after birth, clinical presentation may include cyanosis, severe respiratory distress despite efforts, absence of audible cry, poor air exchange on auscultation, and difficulty with or inability to intubate. If a tracheoesophageal fistula is present, positive pressure ventilation via bag and mask ventilation or esophageal intubation can temporarily help to ventilate the child. Extracorporeal membranous oxygenation may be needed to provide support while a more definitive plan is formulated. Prenatal MRI may assist in diagnosis. An ex utero intrapartum treatment procedure should be undertaken if tracheal agenesis is diagnosed prenatally to secure an airway. Further delineation of the airway includes microlaryngoscopy and bronchoscopy, esophagoscopy, and fine-cut CT imaging of the airway. Tracheal agenesis continues to present a challenge and there are not many good surgical options for reconstruction. Tracheotomy can be attempted. Postnatally diagnosed tracheal agenesis is often lethal. The unavailability of suitable grafting material results in frequent mortality.

Congenital high airway obstruction syndrome deserves special mention. Congenital high airway obstruction syndrome results from tracheal agenesis or larnyngotracheal stenosis/obstruction. Congenital high airway obstruction syndrome can be diagnosed prenatally when ultrasound examination and MRI reveal enlarged hyperechogenic lungs, fluid-filled dilated trachea, flattened or inverted diaphragms, compression of the heart, and sometimes visualization of the obstruction.[20] An ex utero intrapartum treatment procedure can help to secure an airway through a fetal tracheotomy or laryngoscopy and bronchoscopy. Laryngotracheal reconstruction can then be performed.

OTHER RARE ANOMALIES

Tracheal neoplasms are very rare in children. Among the histologic types, both benign and malignant tumors have been identified, including carcinoid, carcinoma, chondroma, hamartoma, hemangioma, microfibrolastic inflammatory tumor, granulosa cell tumor, and lipoblastoma. With endoluminal compression, these tumors can be misinterpreted as symptoms of asthma and recurrent pulmonary infections. Medical treatment with an oral beta-blocker is the first line of treatment for hemangiomas, whereas inflammatory tumors are often treated with nonsteroidal antiinflammatories. Endoluminal or open surgery, consisting of tumor resection or open tracheal resection, are part of the management strategy. Slide tracheoplasty or sleeve resections are commonly used.

SUMMARY

The management of pediatric patients with disorders of the thorax represents a key component of the practice of thoracic surgery. Vascular rings, slings, and tracheobronchial disorders leading to airway and esophageal obstruction are rare but important pathologies. As part of routine clinical practice, the thoracic surgeon will come across patients afflicted with such disorders. A working knowledge of the pathophysiology, diagnosis, and management of these disorders is requisite in the practice of thoracic surgery.

REFERENCES

1. Brenner D, Elliston C, Hall E, et al. Estimated risks of radiation-induced fatal cancer from computed tomography. Am J Roentgenol 2001;176:289–96.
2. Hall E. Lessons we have learned from our children: cancer risks from diagnostic radiology. Pediatr Radiol 2002;32:700–6.
3. Shah R, Mora B, Bacha E, et al. The presentation and management of vascular rings: an otolaryngology perspective. Int J Pediatr Otorhinolaryngol 2007;71:57–62.
4. Kussman B, Geva T, McGowan F. Cardiovascular causes of airway compression. Paediatr Anaesth 2004;14:60–74.
5. McLaren C, Elliott M, Roebuck D. Vascular compression of the airway in children. Paediatr Respir Rev 2008;9:85–94.
6. Tatekawa Y, Tojo T, Hori T, et al. A new technique for treatment of tracheal compression by the innominate artery: external reinforcement with autologous cartilage graft and muscle flap suspension. Pediatr Surg Int 2008;24:431–5.
7. Tsugawa C, Ono Y, Nishijima E, et al. Transection of the innominate artery for tracheomalacia caused by persistent opisthotonus. Pediatr Surg Int 2004;20:55–7.
8. O'Byrne M, Rome N, Santamaria R, et al. Intraprocedural bronchoscopy to prevent bronchial compression during pulmonary artery stent angioplasty. Pediatr Cardiol 2016;37(3):433–41.
9. Hysinger E, Panitch H. Paediatric tracheomalacia. Paediatr Respir Rev 2016;17:9–15.
10. Carden K, Boiselle P, Waltz D, et al. Tracheomalacia and tracheobronchomalacia in children and adults: an in-depth review. Chest 2005;127:984–1005.
11. Boogaard R, Huijsman S, Pijnenburg M, et al. Tracheomalacia and bronchomalacia in children. Chest 2005;128:3391–7.
12. Zopf D, Hollister S, Nelson M, et al. Bioresorbable airway splint created with a three-dimensional printer. N Engl J Med 2013;368:2043–5.
13. Sandu K, Monnier P. Congenital tracheal anomalies. Otolaryngol Clin North Am 2007;40:193–217.
14. Butler C, Speggiorin S, Rijnberg F, et al. Outcomes of slide tracheoplasty in 101 children: a 17-year single-center experience. Cardiovasc Surg 2014;147:1783–90.
15. Grillo H, Wright C, Vlahakes G, et al. Management of congenital tracheal stenosis by means of slide tracheoplasty or resection and reconstruction, with long-term follow-up of growth after slide tracheoplasty. J Thorac Cardiovasc Surg 2002;123:145–52.
16. Noorily M, Farmer D, Belenky W, et al. Congenital tracheal anomalies in the craniosynostosis syndromes. J Pediatr Surg 1999;34:1036–9.
17. Scheid S, Spector A, Luft J. Tracheal cartilaginous sleeve in Crouzon syndrome. Int J Pediatr Otorhinolaryngol 2002;65:147–52.
18. Heimann K, Bartz C, Naami A, et al. Three new cases of congenital agenesis of the trachea. Eur J Pediatr 2007;166:79–82.
19. Floyd J, Campbell D, Dominy D. Agenesis of the trachea. Am Rev Respir Dis 1962;86:557–60.
20. De Groot-van der Mooren M, Haak M, Lakeman P, et al. Tracheal agenesis: approach towards this severe diagnosis. Case report and review of the literature. Eur J Pediatr 2012;171:42.

Esophagectomy After Weight-Reduction Surgery

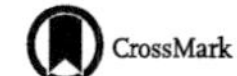

Katy A. Marino, MD, Benny Weksler, MBA, MD*

KEYWORDS

• Esophagectomy • Esophageal adenocarcinoma • Bariatric surgery • Gastric bypass

KEY POINTS

- The incidence of obesity is increasing worldwide.
- Combined with reflux, male sex, and white race, obesity is a known risk factor for esophageal cancer.
- The incidence of esophageal cancer after bariatric surgery is unknown.
- Esophagectomy can be performed after bariatric surgery in many patients.
- There is a paucity of information on the incidence and best approach to esophagectomy after bariatric surgery.

INTRODUCTION

The incidence of esophageal cancer increased more than 350% from the 1970s to the 1990s, mostly because of an increase in the incidence of esophageal adenocarcinoma.[1] Fortunately, this rapid increase in incidence seems to have slowed down in recent years.[2] Half of patients diagnosed with esophageal adenocarcinoma (50%) are obese, smoke cigarettes, or drink alcohol, and up to 87% of patients with esophageal squamous cell carcinoma smoke or drink alcohol.[3] In particular, increases in body mass index are correlated with an increased risk of esophageal adenocarcinoma.[4]

Obesity has become epidemic throughout the world with increasing prevalence on all continents.[5] In 2007, it was estimated that 35% of white men and women, and up to 55% of black women in the United States would be obese by 2010.[6] These predictions have turned out to be surprisingly accurate. The most recent national data on obesity (2011–2014) indicate that the prevalence of obesity among adults in the United States is 36.5%, with a prevalence of 34.5% in non-Hispanic white adults and a prevalence of 56.9% in black women.[7] The number of obese patients who undergo bariatric surgery, primarily Roux-en-Y gastric bypass (RYGB), increased from less than 7000 per year in 1996 to 45,473 in 2001 and seems to have plateaued at 113,000 patients per year in 2010.[8,9] The salutary effects of bariatric surgery are well established.[10–12]

The incidence of esophageal cancer arising after bariatric surgery is unknown. A recent systematic review of the literature found only 11 reported patients with esophageal cancer arising after bariatric surgery, and only seven underwent esophagectomy after bariatric surgery.[13] Our own literature review identified nine additional published cases, and we have personally performed

Disclosures: B. Weksler is a Proctor for Intuitive Surgery and a Consultant for Bard.

Division of Thoracic Surgery, University of Tennessee Health Science Center, 1325 Eastmoreland Avenue, Suite #460, Memphis, TN 38104, USA
* Corresponding author.
E-mail address: bweksler@uthsc.edu

Thorac Surg Clin 28 (2018) 53–58
https://doi.org/10.1016/j.thorsurg.2017.08.006

esophagectomy on two patients after bariatric surgery (**Table 1**).

Currently 95.7% of bariatric procedures are performed laparoscopically and the most common procedures worldwide are RYGB (45%), sleeve gastrectomy (SG; 37%), and band gastroplasty (BG; 10%).[14] Each of these procedures offers challenges for the surgeon during esophagectomy.

TECHNICAL CONSIDERATIONS

We briefly describe each of the common, bariatric procedures to provide an understanding of the surgical anatomy after each procedure as it relates to esophagectomy.

Roux-en-Y Gastric Bypass

The technique for laparoscopic RYGB has been described and is uniform.[15] Briefly, a small proximal gastric pouch is created by completely dividing it from the rest of the stomach. Commonly, a biliary-pancreatic limb is created 50 cm from the ligament of Treitz and is anastomosed to the Roux limb with a length of approximately 75 to 100 cm. The Roux limb is positioned either in the retrocolic and retrogastric position or in the antecolic and antegastric position.[16] The Roux limb is then anastomosed to the proximal gastric pouch (**Fig. 1**). It is important to remember that during RYGB in the retrocolic fashion, there are three mesenteric defects that are closed and need to be addressed during esophagectomy: (1) a defect in the transverse mesocolon just lateral to the ligament of Treitz, (2) the mesentery of the small bowel, and (3) Petersen defect (the space behind the Roux limb). In antecolic RYGB only the mesentery of the small bowel and Petersen defect are closed.

When performing an esophagectomy after RYGB, the stomach is usually suitable for use as a conduit (**Fig. 2**). The gastroepiploic arcade is usually undisturbed, and an adequate length of mobile gastric conduit is obtained, even for a cervical anastomosis. There is one report of a divided gastroepiploic arcade after RYGB in a patient

Table 1
Additional patients who underwent esophagectomy after a bariatric procedure

Study Author	Number of Patients	Age (y)	Prior Bariatric Procedure	Time Between Bariatric Procedure and Esophagectomy	Histology	Esophageal Replacement Conduit	Follow-up[a] (mo)
Allen et al,[21] 2004	2	54, 50	RYGB	21 y, 14 y	EAC	Jejunum, stomach	13,[b] 72
Trincado et al,[22] 2005	1	52	BG followed by RYGB	5 y	EAC	Stomach	12
Nguyen et al,[19] 2006	1	56	RYGB	5 y	EAC	Stomach	3.5
Melstrom et al,[30] 2008	2	55, 58	RYGB	2 mo, 3 y	EAC, HGD	Stomach	60, 24
Kuruba et al,[39] 2009	1	45	RYGB	20 mo	EAC	Stomach	NR
Rossidis et al,[17] 2014	5	57	RYGB	NR	EAC	Stomach (n = 4) Colon (n = 1)	NR
Boules et al,[33] 2016	2	40, 50	BG	NR	Achalasia	Stomach	36
Ellison et al,[18] 2016	2	66, 49	RYGB	3 mo, 4 mo	EAC	Stomach	19, 36
Weksler and Sullivan,[35] 2017[c]	2	53, 58	RYGB and BG	3 y, 5 y	EAC	Stomach	12, 14

Abbreviations: BG, band gastroplasty; EAC, esophageal adenocarcinoma; HGD, high-grade dysplasia; NR, not reported.
[a] Except as noted, all patients were alive at the last recorded follow-up.
[b] This patient died 13 months after esophagectomy.
[c] Our previously unpublished results.

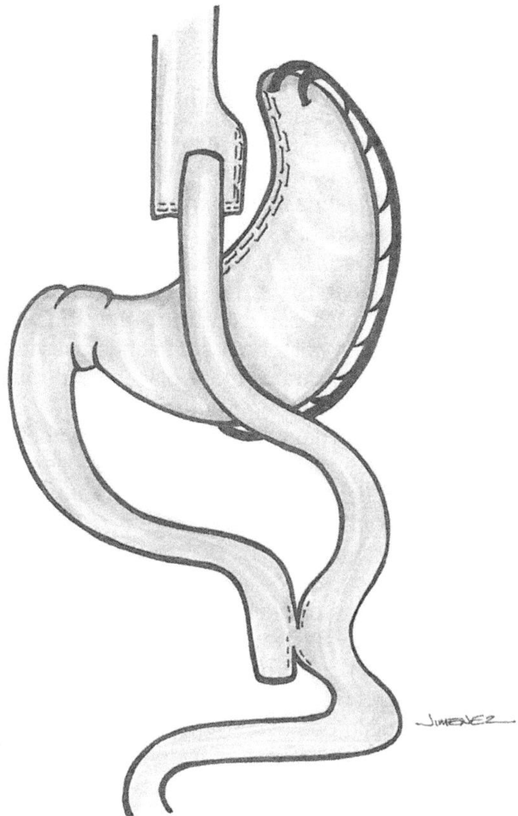

Fig. 1. Schematic depicting the anatomy of the esophagus, stomach, and jejunum after an RYBG. (*From* Rossidis G, Browning R, Hochwald SN, et al. Minimally invasive esophagectomy is safe in patients with previous gastric bypass. Surg Obes Relat Dis 2014;10:97; with permission.)

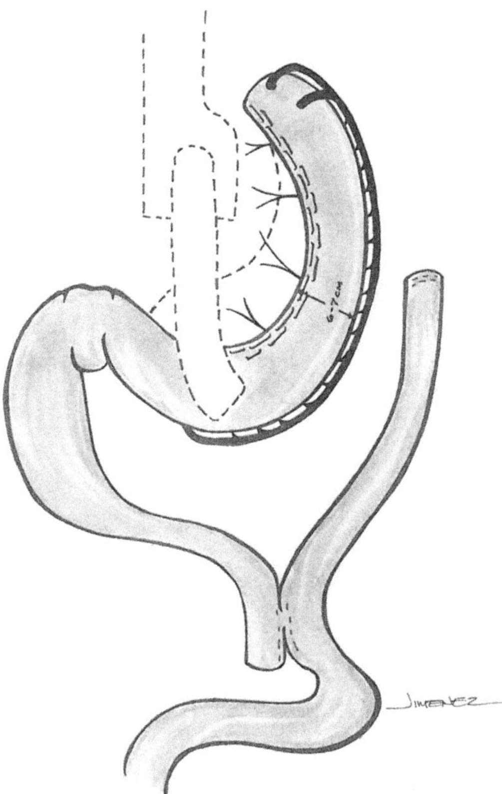

Fig. 2. Creation of the gastric conduit from the remnant stomach during esophagectomy after RYGB. (*From* Rossidis G, Browning R, Hochwald SN, et al. Minimally invasive esophagectomy is safe in patients with previous gastric bypass. Surg Obes Relat Dis 2014;10:98; with permission.)

requiring esophagectomy; this patient required a colonic interposition.[17] It is prudent to prepare patients with prior bariatric procedures for the possibility of a colon interposition rather than an esophagectomy with the stomach as the replacement conduit by performing colonoscopy, computed tomography angiography of the mesenteric vessels, and bowel preparation preoperatively.

During esophagectomy, the anatomy of the Roux limb should be recognized as antecolic or retrocolic. The gastrohepatic ligament is dissected and the left gastric vessels are identified. The Roux limb is divided a few centimeters below the gastric pouch and it can be used as a handle. A celiac node dissection is performed, and the left gastric vessels divided. The gastric remnant is then mobilized completely with care taken to preserve the gastroepiploic arcade, and a narrow gastric tube is fashioned. The Roux limb can then be resected, reanastomosed to the biliary pancreatic limb, or used to create a jejunostomy, which is our preference (**Fig. 3**).[17–19] Pyloroplasty is controversial in this context, and we prefer not to perform it. Finally, the distal esophagus is mobilized into the mediastinum, and the gastric conduit sutured to the gastric pouch.

Because many patients have a lower esophageal or gastroesophageal junction tumor, we prefer a chest anastomosis. The thoracic portion of the procedure and the intrathoracic anastomosis has been described.[20] It is worth noting that the abdominal portion of the procedure can be done either with traditional laparotomy[21,22] or using minimally invasive techniques.[17,19]

Laparoscopic Gastric Sleeve Resection

Gastric sleeve resection is becoming more popular and currently 37% of patients who undergo a bariatric procedure undergo SG.[14] SG involves the resection of the greater curvature of the

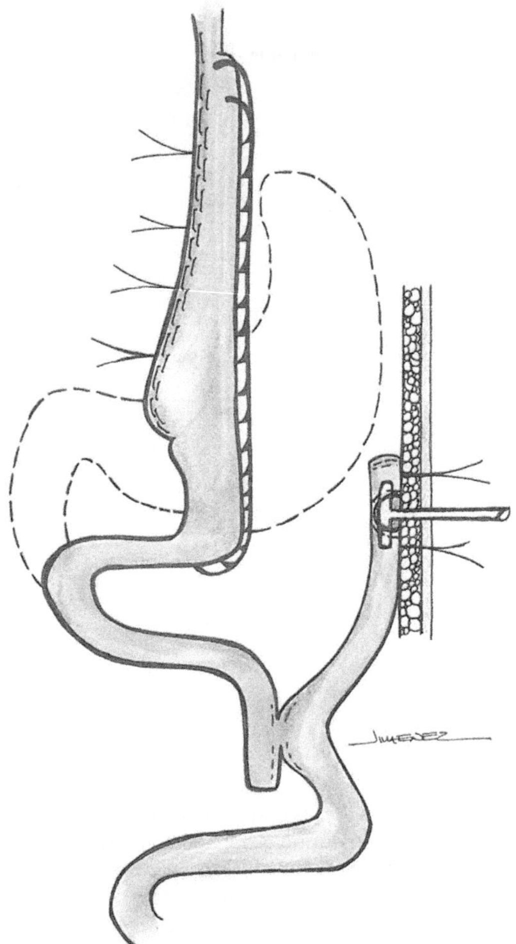

Fig. 3. A feeding jejunostomy placed in the Roux limb after esophagectomy. (*From* Rossidis G, Browning R, Hochwald SN, et al. Minimally invasive esophagectomy is safe in patients with previous gastric bypass. Surg Obes Relat Dis 2014;10:98; with permission.)

stomach, starting 4 to 6 cm from the pylorus, creating a narrow gastric tube over a bougie, parallel to the lesser curvature, preserving the left and right gastric vessels.[23] The gastroepiploic arcade is sacrificed during the procedure or is completely detached from the stomach. There are no reports of patients undergoing esophagectomy after SG, and there is only one reported case of esophageal cancer after SG.[24] We speculate that the stomach would not provide much length for an Ivor Lewis or Mckeown esophagectomy and that alternative conduit should be considered. We believe that the best approach for these patients would be resection of the remaining stomach and esophagus, with colon interposition and Roux-en-Y colojejunal anastomosis.

Band Gastroplasty

BG is not as commonly performed as RYGB or SG. There are two types of bands that are applied in BG: an adjustable band, which is more commonly used today; and a vertical band that does not allow for adjustments. The adjustable band is placed just below the gastroesophageal junction creating a small gastric pouch.[25] Usually the greater curvature is undisturbed. The band has a port, which is placed subcutaneously in the abdominal wall to allow injection of saline and band adjustment. Often the anterior wall of the stomach is used to cover the band in one or more places, and this needs to be undone to remove the band.

Vertical-banded gastroplasty is less commonly performed today. It involves creating a narrow gastric pouch based on the lesser curvature and placing a polymeric silicone band (Lap Band, Apollo endosurgery, Austin, TX) around the lower part of the pouch.[26] Older techniques used other materials, such as crystalline polypropylene with high-density polyethylene (Marlex, C,R, Bard, Murray Hill, NJ), to create a band.[27] As with adjustable band placement, the greater curvature is usually undisturbed.

There are reported cases of esophageal cancer after BG, but surprisingly there have been no reports of esophagectomy for cancer after BG as a stand-alone bariatric procedure.[21,28–32] Boules reported on two patients who had esophagectomy for end-stage achalasia after vertical-banded gastroplasty.[33] To perform esophagectomy after BG using either technique, the band must be removed, which may be difficult, because bands may erode into the stomach with time. After the band is removed, the esophagectomy proceeds with the mobilization of the stomach and creation of a traditional gastric tube supplied by the right gastroepiploic arcade. Usually there is enough conduit length to replace the esophagus. In our case of a patient with esophageal cancer after a prior vertical-banded gastroplasty (detailed in **Table 1**), we followed the previously mentioned steps and did not have difficulty with conduit length or viability.

OTHER CONSIDERATIONS

Approach to Perform the Esophagectomy: Open, Minimally Invasive, or Robotic?

Minimally invasive esophagectomy has been shown to improve morbidity, but not operative mortality, when compared with open esophagectomy.[34] It is unclear if minimally invasive esophagectomy improves long-term survival. Our work suggests that there are no differences in survival in patients who undergo minimally invasive as compared with open esophagectomy.[35] There are several reports of successful minimally invasive approaches to esophagectomy after bariatric surgery,[17–19] and minimally invasive esophagectomy can be performed if the surgeon is comfortable with the technique.

Should Patients Undergoing Bariatric Procedures be Screened for Esophageal Cancer?

There are no preoperative screening guidelines for upper endoscopy in patients without upper gastrointestinal symptoms who are preparing to undergo bariatric surgery. In a recent report, two patients who underwent intraoperative anastomotic surveillance during laparoscopic RYGB were found to have biopsy-proven esophageal adenocarcinoma.[18] Because the endoscopy occurred after the gastrojejunal anastomosis was created, the surgeons completed the bariatric procedure in both patients, who later underwent laparoscopic transhiatal esophagectomy using the gastric remnant as a conduit to create a cervical esophagogastrostomy. Schirmer and colleagues[36] performed upper endoscopy on 536 patients undergoing a bariatric procedure and found that 4.9% had a change in management, most commonly placement of a gastrostomy tube in patients with gastritis. Through this screening, Schirmer identified one patient with high-grade dysplasia who had an esophagectomy, but did not find any patients with esophageal cancer. In a series of 448 morbidly obese patients who underwent preoperative upper endoscopy, Loewen and colleagues[37] found that findings from the upper endoscopy changed their preoperative management in 18% of patients and changed their surgical approach in one patient. The authors did not detect any esophageal adenocarcinoma. Humphreys and colleagues[38] performed endoscopy before bariatric surgery in 371 patients. More than half of the patients had an abnormal upper endoscopy; most had a hiatal hernia. The authors detected esophageal adenocarcinoma in two patients, and one of the patients underwent esophagectomy. Although controversial, we believe that there is enough evidence in the literature to justify upper endoscopy in all patients before bariatric surgery, in part, because upper endoscopy is a simple procedure with few complications.

SUMMARY

With more than 113,000 bariatric procedures performed yearly in the United States, esophageal surgeons can expect to manage patients with esophageal cancer after bariatric procedures. Knowledge of the patient's anatomy and the type of bariatric procedure that was performed is crucial to the success of the esophagectomy. The stomach of most patients can be used as a conduit during esophagectomy, although patients who have undergone an SG procedure are the exception. The true incidence of esophageal cancer after bariatric procedures and the number of patients who undergo esophagectomy after a bariatric procedure are unknown. Larger studies on the subject may provide information on short- and long-term outcomes.

ACKNOWLEDGMENTS

The authors acknowledge Shannon Wyszomierski, PhD for expert scientific editorial review.

REFERENCES

1. Devesa SS, Blot WJ, Fraumeni JF Jr. Changing patterns in the incidence of esophageal and gastric carcinoma in the United States. Cancer 1998; 83(10):2049–53.
2. Hur C, Miller M, Kong CY, et al. Trends in esophageal adenocarcinoma incidence and mortality. Cancer 2013;119(6):1149–58.
3. Vaughan TL, Davis S, Kristal A, et al. Obesity, alcohol, and tobacco as risk factors for cancers of the esophagus and gastric cardia: adenocarcinoma versus squamous cell carcinoma. Cancer Epidemiol Biomarkers Prev 1995;4(2):85–92.
4. Chow WH, Blot WJ, Vaughan TL, et al. Body mass index and risk of adenocarcinomas of the esophagus and gastric cardia. J Natl Cancer Inst 1998; 90(2):150–5.
5. James PT, Leach R, Kalamara E, et al. The worldwide obesity epidemic. Obes Res 2001;9(Suppl 4): 228S–33S.
6. Wang YC, Colditz GA, Kuntz KM. Forecasting the obesity epidemic in the aging U.S. population. Obesity (Silver Spring) 2007;15(11):2855–65.
7. Ogden CL, Carroll MD, Fryar CD, et al. Prevalence of obesity among adults and youth: United States, 2011-2014. NCHS Data Brief 2015;(219):1–8.
8. Livingston EH. Procedure incidence and in-hospital complication rates of bariatric surgery in the United States. Am J Surg 2004;188(2):105–10.
9. Livingston EH. The incidence of bariatric surgery has plateaued in the U.S. Am J Surg 2010;200(3): 378–85.
10. Sjostrom L, Narbro K, Sjostrom CD, et al. Effects of bariatric surgery on mortality in Swedish obese subjects. N Engl J Med 2007;357(8):741–52.
11. Sjostrom L, Gummesson A, Sjostrom CD, et al. Effects of bariatric surgery on cancer incidence in

obese patients in Sweden (Swedish Obese Subjects Study): a prospective, controlled intervention trial. Lancet Oncol 2009;10(7):653–62.
12. Schauer PR, Kashyap SR, Wolski K, et al. Bariatric surgery versus intensive medical therapy in obese patients with diabetes. N Engl J Med 2012; 366(17):1567–76.
13. Scozzari G, Trapani R, Toppino M, et al. Esophagogastric cancer after bariatric surgery: systematic review of the literature. Surg Obes Relat Dis 2013;9(1): 133–42.
14. Angrisani L, Santonicola A, Iovino P, et al. Bariatric surgery worldwide 2013. Obes Surg 2015;25(10): 1822–32.
15. Schauer PR, Ikramuddin S, Gourash W, et al. Outcomes after laparoscopic Roux-en-Y gastric bypass for morbid obesity. Ann Surg 2000;232(4):515–29.
16. Steele KE, Prokopowicz GP, Magnuson T, et al. Laparoscopic antecolic Roux-en-Y gastric bypass with closure of internal defects leads to fewer internal hernias than the retrocolic approach. Surg Endosc 2008;22(9):2056–61.
17. Rossidis G, Browning R, Hochwald SN, et al. Minimally invasive esophagectomy is safe in patients with previous gastric bypass. Surg Obes Relat Dis 2014;10(1):95–100.
18. Ellison HB, Parker DM, Horsley RD, et al. Laparoscopic transhiatal esophagectomy for esophageal adenocarcinoma identified at laparoscopic Roux-en-Y gastric bypass. Int J Surg Case Rep 2016;25: 179–83.
19. Nguyen NT, Tran CL, Gelfand DV, et al. Laparoscopic and thoracoscopic Ivor Lewis esophagectomy after Roux-en-Y gastric bypass. Ann Thorac Surg 2006;82(5):1910–3.
20. Luketich JD, Pennathur A, Awais O, et al. Outcomes after minimally invasive esophagectomy: review of over 1000 patients. Ann Surg 2012;256(1):95–103.
21. Allen JW, Leeman MF, Richardson JD. Esophageal carcinoma following bariatric procedures. JSLS 2004;8(4):372–5.
22. Trincado MT, del Olmo JC, Garcia Castano J, et al. Gastric pouch carcinoma after gastric bypass for morbid obesity. Obes Surg 2005;15(8):1215–7.
23. Cottam D, Qureshi FG, Mattar SG, et al. Laparoscopic sleeve gastrectomy as an initial weight-loss procedure for high-risk patients with morbid obesity. Surg Endosc 2006;20(6):859–63.
24. Scheepers AF, Schoon EJ, Nienhuijs SW. Esophageal carcinoma after sleeve gastrectomy. Surg Obes Relat Dis 2011;7(4):e11–2.
25. Ren CJ. Controversies in bariatric surgery: evidence-based discussions on laparoscopic adjustable gastric banding. J Gastrointest Surg 2004;8(4):396–7 [discussion: 404–5].
26. Lonroth H, Dalenback J, Haglind E, et al. Vertical banded gastroplasty by laparoscopic technique in the treatment of morbid obesity. Surg Laparosc Endosc 1996;6(2):102–7.
27. Suter M, Jayet C, Jayet A. Vertical banded gastroplasty: long-term results comparing three different techniques. Obes Surg 2000;10(1):41–6 [discussion: 47].
28. Snook KL, Ritchie JD. Carcinoma of esophagus after adjustable gastric banding. Obes Surg 2003;13(5): 800–2.
29. Hackert T, Dietz M, Tjaden C, et al. Band erosion with gastric cancer. Obes Surg 2004;14(4):559–61.
30. Melstrom LG, Bentrem DJ, Salvino MJ, et al. Adenocarcinoma of the gastroesophageal junction after bariatric surgery. Am J Surg 2008;196(1):135–8.
31. Korswagen LA, Schrama JG, Bruins Slot W, et al. Adenocarcinoma of the lower esophagus after placement of a gastric band. Obes Surg 2009; 19(3):389–92.
32. Stauffer JA, Mathew J, Odell JA. Esophageal adenocarcinoma after laparoscopic gastric band placement for obesity. Dis Esophagus 2011;24(1):E8–10.
33. Boules M, Corcelles R, Zelisko A, et al. Achalasia after bariatric surgery. J Laparoendosc Adv Surg Tech A 2016;26(6):428–32.
34. Biere SS, van Berge Henegouwen MI, Maas KW, et al. Minimally invasive versus open oesophagectomy for patients with oesophageal cancer: a multicentre, open-label, randomised controlled trial. Lancet 2012;379(9829):1887–92.
35. Weksler B, Sullivan JL. Survival after esophagectomy: a propensity-matched study of different surgical approaches. Ann Thorac Surg 2017. [Epub ahead of print].
36. Schirmer B, Erenoglu C, Miller A. Flexible endoscopy in the management of patients undergoing Roux-en-Y gastric bypass. Obes Surg 2002;12(5): 634–8.
37. Loewen M, Giovanni J, Barba C. Screening endoscopy before bariatric surgery: a series of 448 patients. Surg Obes Relat Dis 2008;4(6):709–12.
38. Humphreys LM, Meredith H, Morgan J, et al. Detection of asymptomatic adenocarcinoma at endoscopy prior to gastric banding justifies routine endoscopy. Obes Surg 2012;22(4):594–6.
39. Kuruba R, Jawad M, Karl RC, et al. Technique of resection of esophageal adenocarcinoma after Roux-en-Y gastric bypass and literature review of esophagogastric tumors after bariatric procedures. Surg Obes Relat Dis 2009;5(5):576–81.

Thoracic Surgery Considerations in the Mentally Ill or Handicapped Patient

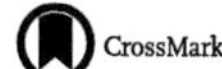

Anthony B. Mozer, MD, MBA[a], James E. Speicher, MD[b], Carlos J. Anciano, MD[b,c,*]

KEYWORDS

• Increasing prevalence • Perioperative care • Increased morbidity • Ethical implications

KEY POINTS

- Mentally ill and handicapped are an increasing patient group with added morbidity and mortality for thoracic interventions.
- Surgical indications, oncologic principles, and infectious considerations should remain the same.
- Technical procedure details and aggressive perioperative management impact outcomes.
- Patient functional status, caregiver capacity, and idiosyncrasies of baseline mental illness must be incorporated in the surgical algorithm and considerations.
- Multispecialty case discussion, incorporating ethical implications of care and goals, is to be incorporated in the complex informed consent process.

 **Video content accompanies this article at http://www.thoracic.theclinics.com.**

INTRODUCTION

Thoracic surgeons can anticipate caring for patients with an increasing burden of comorbid conditions and chronic disease. As a result of improved preventative care, medical treatment, and surgical intervention for acute illness, disease-specific mortality continues to decline more rapidly than the prevalence of chronic disease, worldwide.[1] Over the past 25 years, there has been a staggering 91.8% increase in the global burden of disease specifically attributable to dementia, as measured in years lived with disability. Of the estimated 44.4 million people worldwide with dementia, most are older than the age of 65, increasing the likelihood for comorbid cardiopulmonary disease requiring thoracic intervention in this population.[2] Including mood, behavioral, and substance abuse disorders, more than one-fifth (21.2%) of global years lived with disability is now linked to mental illness.[1] An estimated 154 million individuals worldwide live with intellectual impairment, one-third of whom exhibit moderate (IQ <50) to profound debility.[1] Patients

Disclosure Statement: There are no disclosures or conflicts of interest.

[a] General Surgery Resident, Department of Surgery, East Carolina University, 600 Moye Boulevard, Greenville, NC 27834, USA; [b] Thoracic and Foregut Surgery, Department of Cardiovascular Sciences, East Carolina University, 115 Heart Drive, Greenville, NC 27834, USA; [c] Minimally Invasive Thoracic Surgery, Department of Cardiovascular Sciences, East Carolina University, 115 Heart Drive, Greenville, NC 27834, USA
* Corresponding author. Minimally Invasive Thoracic Surgery, Department of Cardiovascular Sciences, East Carolina University, 115 Heart Drive, Greenville, NC 27834.
E-mail address: ancianoc14@ecu.edu

Thorac Surg Clin 28 (2018) 59–68
https://doi.org/10.1016/j.thorsurg.2017.08.007

with neurologic, cognitive, or behavioral debility present a unique set of circumstances to the thoracic surgeon as a function of their disease and because of complexities associated with their support system and living environment. Here, we outline important considerations in managing the complexities of the increasingly prevalent mentally ill or handicapped thoracic surgery patient population. In the interest of illustrating the complex and variant clinical situations this patient population presents, we follow with real-life scenarios in our practice. We concentrate discussions on technical aspects and considerations particular to these states. The standard surgical indications, approaches, and management of the thoracic pathology remain the same. Antibiotic management for pneumonia, surgical resection of an early lung cancer, or plication of a paralyzed diaphragm are not the focus, but the added considerations to be had.

RESPIRATORY FAILURE AND AIRWAY MANAGEMENT

Case 1

MD is a 55-year-old bedbound woman with lower extremity contractures caused by cerebral palsy who developed a spontaneous, left-sided pneumothorax while living at a long-term acute care facility. This followed an inpatient stay for care of multidrug-resistant organism infection of chronic decubitus ulcers. She was initially managed at a regional hospital with multiple chest tubes for a 2-week period and was transferred to our tertiary care center for thoracic surgery evaluation and management because of concern for a bronchopleural fistula. After a trial of conservative management and under suspicion for iatrogenic lung injury (**Figs. 1** and **2**), she was taken to the operating room for video-assisted thoracoscopic wedge resection, partial pleurectomy, and mechanical pleurodesis. The patient's severe lower extremity contractures prevented normal positioning with a beanbag on the operating room table, so she was positioned with her legs supine and her thorax elevated with pillows. She was stabilized with gel pads surrounding her entire body to hold her in position and protect from inappropriate body contortion and further damage to her pre-existing decubitus ulcers. Postoperatively, she had difficulty with management of secretions and with suspected pneumonia, resulting in desaturations and requiring bronchial hygiene maneuvers including therapeutic bronchoscopy, but was ultimately able to be discharged back to her facility under the care of her sister and caregivers (**Fig. 3**, Video 1).

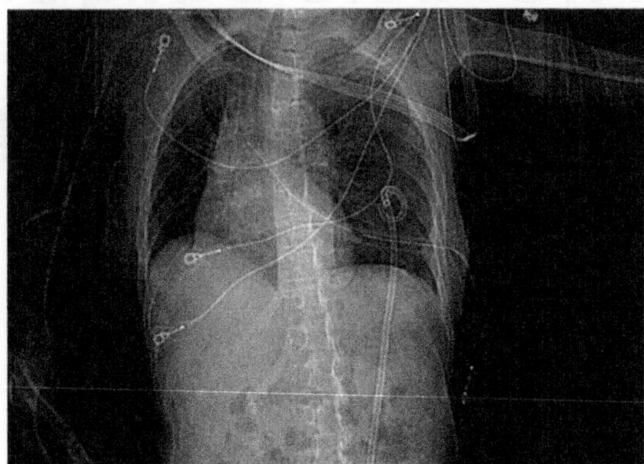

Fig. 1. Admission computed tomography scout with multiple drains and distorted chest anatomy.

Discussion

Respiratory complications continue to represent the primary morbidity in thoracic interventions. The value of pulmonary toilet, early ambulation,

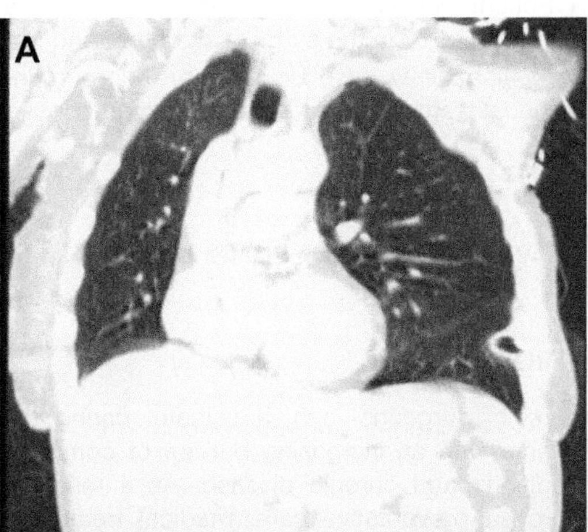

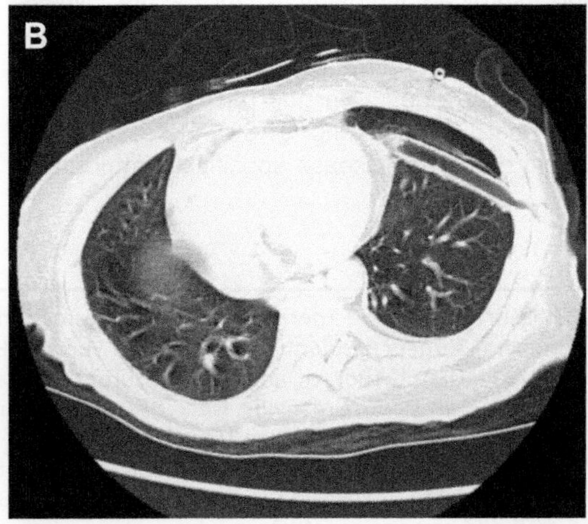

Fig. 2. Iatrogenic lung injury. (*A*) Entrance injury. (*B*) Parenchymal trajectory.

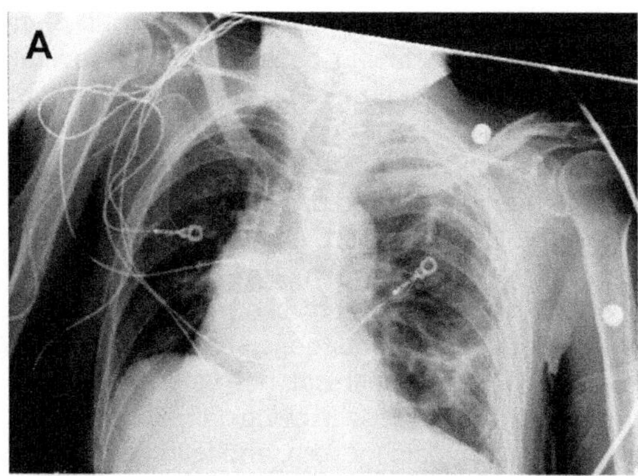

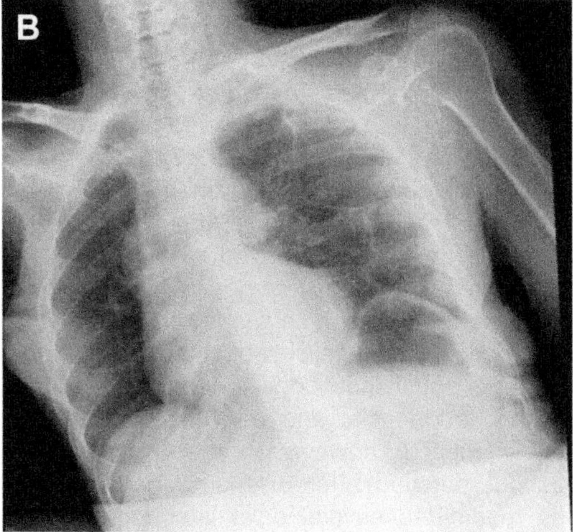

Fig. 3. Postoperative and follow-up chest radiograph. (*A*) Postoperative chest radiograph. (*B*) Outpatient follow-up chest radiograph.

body position change, and optimization of West ventilation perfusion zones is paramount in the treatment, and more importantly, the prevention of respiratory complications in the mentally ill and handicapped population. Limitations in performance capacity and understanding of simple maneuvers may make the use of incentive spirometry, flutter valve, and other forms of intermittent vibratory lung expansion and cough support mechanism less effective. As a result, close partnership with nursing and respiratory therapy staff in providing directed chest therapies including vibratory beds, vests, assisted frequent positional changes, and thoracic percussion, coupled with secretion management strategies as nasotracheal suctioning becomes critical to successful convalescence. We favor aggressive bronchoscopic toilet, at times more than once daily, using pediatric-sized bronchoscopes with adult-size working channels to permit a less traumatic nasal approach for invasive secretion management. This can be performed effectively in seconds to minutes, have a clear impact on ventilation states, and is well-tolerated using minimal or no sedation. We favor preprocedure lidocaine nebulization and local topical anesthetics with glotic-tracheal instillation for the nasal approach, prompting a natural cough reflex and secretion clearance that aids in the toilet process. Avoidance of sedation minimizes the postprocedure downtime that often leads to aspiration of endogenous oronasal secretions and poor airway protection that undermines the initial purpose of the bronchoscopy. We advocate for frequent culture of respiratory secretions, because nursing homes and specialized care facilities harbor idiosyncratic respiratory flora. It is critical to intervene well before lung “white-out” in these patients. Chest radiographs tend to lag behind the true clinical status of the airways in this population, and spinal deformities, rotated films caused by body morphology, anatomic contractions, and poor voluntary inspiratory effort on command diminish the quality and reliability of the images.

Although often viewed with trepidation by family members, early tracheostomy placement accommodates considerably more effective and less traumatic invasive airway toilet. Prevention of secondary pressure sores cannot be underestimated. The potential lesions are not limited to the hardware on the skin but internal tracheal and proximal mainstem mucosal ulcerations and erosions. In planning for tracheostomy, body habitus is carefully considered for length and for pressure point establishment. The altered positioning caused by contractions or cervical mobility limitations in this population impacts the internal positioning of the tracheostomy tube profile, and we favor an open approach for placement of stay sutures and evaluation of pressure points within the airway. In contrast to other populations, the need for a surgical airway may be long term, and careful assessment prevents internal ulcerations, dreaded fistulous complications, and valve and flap-like effects that result from distal intermittent obstructions caused by positioning toward the airway walls. We recommend evaluating for innominate artery position, because variance in the shape of the thoracic cavity may unexpectedly alter its position. Furthermore, many of these patients present with subclinical hypothyroidism, and thyroid enlargement with wide isthmus is often encountered. A frequent cause of reconsultation and patient transfer back to hospital once discharged, we resect the isthmus and lateralize the lobes away from the tracheostomy tube to minimize intermittent bleeds from glandular erosions. Finally, temporary stay sutures limit tracheostomy dislodgement and pull out, a clear risk in the mentally ill patient population in the early postoperative period, and allow for any necessary exchange before a mature tract has developed.

Enteral access for nutrition and medication may be maintained with elective nasogastric access at the time of the index operation. Percutaneous endoscopic gastrostomy is a useful adjunct in many cases. To avoid a vicious spiral of aspirations, pneumonias, frequent readmissions, and steady medical decline, we advocate for careful attention to several seemingly trivial technical details. During endoscopy, it is important to observe mindfully for esophageal tortuosity and cricopharyngeal bars and perform close evaluation of the gastroesophageal junction (GEJ) valve mechanism and the intra-abdominal esophageal length under gastric distention. Patulous valves and small hiatal hernias should prompt a more distal antral placement of the gastrostomy that allows for easy fluoroscopic conversion to a gastrojejunal tube. This allows for enteral feeding access with diminished aspiration risks in this patient frequently bed ridden or in recliners, while maintaining gastric access for decompression and medication access. In the patient presenting with a large hiatal hernia a jejunal access is favored, with a short laparoscopic low-pressure pneumoperitoneum placement. Although they do not prevent dislodgement, the effects of self-removal are mitigated with the use of percutaneous T-fasteners. A laparoscopic approach to gastrostomy access allows for a more robust and enduring gastropexy. The close apposition of the stomach to the abdominal wall can thus be maintained such that dislodgment is amenable to endoscopic rescue. Physiologic tolerance to pneumoperitoneum, previous surgical interventions, chronic body and limb contractions, spine deformities, and other alterations of abdominal phenotype may limit port placement and favor an open approach. Abdominal imaging is recommended in aid of surgical planning in these cases. To minimize the consequences of percutaneous endoscopic gastrostomy removal including gross peritoneal contamination, nursing sign outs and evaluations are to include the height of the gastrostomy tubing at the skin and holster to monitor for changes. Abdominal soft binders also offer some barrier to prevent patient access to the site.

BENIGN FOREGUT DISEASE

Case 2

AH is a 59-year-old woman who does not use tobacco or alcohol and lives in an assisted-living facility in a small town because of an unspecified cognitive disability. She initially presented to a regional medical center for evaluation after an accidental fall, inducing chest pain and several rib fractures. At the time of presentation, she was noted to have an episode of hemoptysis, and a history of peptic ulcer disease was noted for which she had been prescribed daily proton-pump inhibitors (PPI). On admission, she was deemed suitable to make her own medical decisions, but identified her sister, whom she did not live with, as a surrogate. She was observed overnight and discharged back to her residence with instructions to increase her PPI dose to twice daily, discontinue use of nonsteroidals for pain, and follow up with a primary care provider. In the subsequent 3 weeks, she was re-evaluated and discharged from the same regional emergency department, twice for hemoptysis or hematemesis and once for cough and mid-thoracic back pain, after plain films showed no acute abnormality. She was then seen in the emergency department three times over 3 months for behavioral outbursts increasing in severity until being admitted for inpatient psychiatric treatment of severe depression with psychotic features. After an episode of hematemesis as an inpatient, surgical consultation was obtained and an upper endoscopy performed. Marked gastritis, duodenitis, and a 5-cm hiatal hernia were identified; however, further management was not pursued after discharge because she was readmitted several days later for bacterial pneumonia, which required management in the intensive care unit. She was seen in the emergency department on three more occasions for respiratory symptoms, behavioral changes, and falls until a fourth presentation for hematemesis, melena, and abdominal pain prompted a computed tomography scan. This was concerning for ischemic bowel, prompting immediate transfer to the acute care surgery service at our tertiary center (**Fig. 4**, Video 2). Upper endoscopy, laparotomy with hiatal hernia repair, and gastropexy were performed with intraoperative assistance by the general thoracic service. She was managed through a difficult 8-week hospital course and has been seen in follow-up with a small (<2 cm) radiologic recurrence of her hiatal hernia, which was asymptomatic.

Case 3

SS is a 62-year-old woman with a history of dementia and schizophrenia who presented from an assisted-living facility to an outside hospital with abdominal pain, nausea, and vomiting. A computed tomography scan was performed in the emergency department demonstrating an intrathoracic stomach with organomesenteric

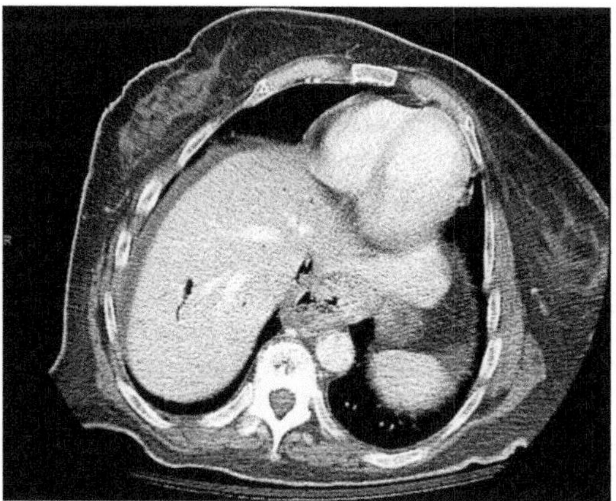

Fig. 4. Incarcerated paraesophageal hernia with ischemia and pneumobilia.

and organoaxial volvulus. Before bringing the patient to the operating room, nasogastric decompression was attempted but unable to be tolerated and she was taken for laparotomy by a general surgeon at the outlying hospital. A laparoscopic approach was attempted and converted to laparotomy, with failure to reduce the gastric volvulus, secondarily resulting in a devascularizing iatrogenic injury to the transverse colon mesentery, which required immediate resection. Subsequently, the patient was transferred to the general surgery service at our tertiary center and admitted to the surgical intensive care unit for resuscitation, ventilatory management, and definitive therapy. The patient's son, living out of state, was identified as the primary health care power of attorney and medical decision-maker because of the patient's state of incapacity. The thoracic surgery service was consulted, imaging was repeated (**Fig. 5**, Video 3), and she was taken to the operating room for temporizing endoscopic reduction and gastric detorsion under fluoroscopic guidance, performed the following day (Video 4). Intraoperative findings were significant for evidence of multiple linear gastric erosions (Cameron lesions). After resuscitation and nasogastric decompression over 72 hours, she was taken for definitive repair including laparoscopic lysis of adhesions, reduction of volvulus with hiatal hernia repair, and gastropexy (Video 5). Following convalescence for 1 month on the surgical unit secondary to prolonged ileus, dysphagia, and psychiatric debility, she was discharged to her living facility in good condition. She has been seen in follow-up with return to baseline function and plans for annual surveillance with barium swallow and pulmonary function testing (**Fig. 6**).

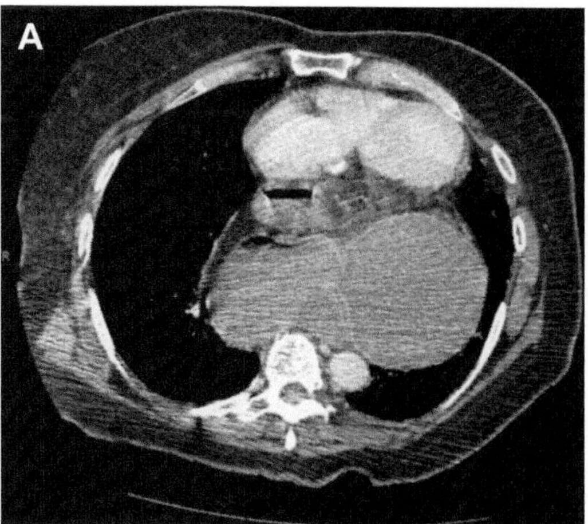

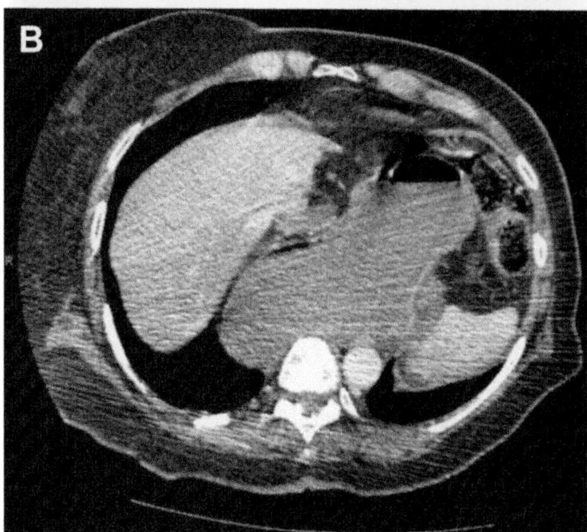

Fig. 5. Computed tomography giant paraesophageal hernia with gastric volvulus. (*A*) Incarcerated intrathoracic stomach with anterior cardiac compression. (*B*) Transhiatal distended gastric body compressing antroduodenal outflow against right crura.

Discussion

As illustrated in the previous vignettes, patients with mental illness and foregut disease present additional challenges to the thoracic surgeon in the diagnosis of disease and in determining the role for and approach to emergency surgery. Twenty percent of adults undergoing routine upper endoscopy are found to have hiatal hernia, with incidence increasing with age.[3] The contribution of hiatal hernia to gastroesophageal reflux disease (GERD) and the findings caused by Cameron lesions, from occult anemia to overt gastrointestinal bleeding, have been well-documented.[4,5] Even in the average patient, diagnosis remains difficult because the pathophysiology and process of this disease is not always appreciated in the broader medical community, the presentation is often variable, and patients may be asymptomatic

A

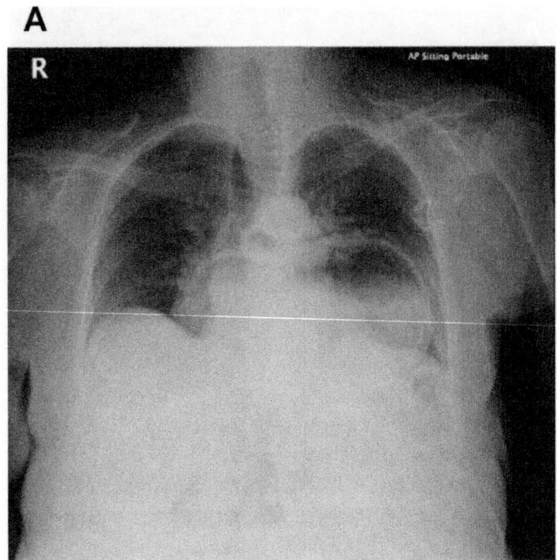

B

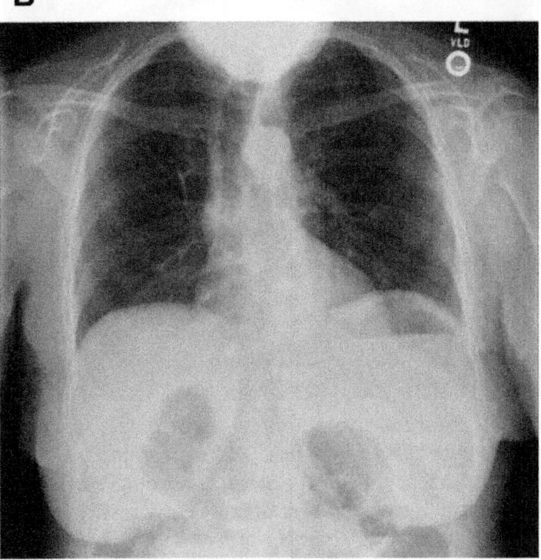

Fig. 6. Preoperative and postoperative chest radiograph in gastric volvulus. (*A*) Preoperative intrathoracic stomach. (*B*) Postoperative subdiaphragmatic stomach.

and never seek evaluation. The development of a giant hiatal hernia is considered progression of the type I, or sliding, hernia with migration of the stomach and sometimes other abdominal viscera into the mediastinum.[6] Type II, III, and IV hernias are considered indications for surgery because of the unpredictable and catastrophic complications of disease including volvulus, obstruction, and strangulation, which may all precipitate morbidity and mortality from perforation or frank necrosis.[6] Nonelective repair in propensity-matched patient populations carries an odds ratio of 1.67 and 2.74 for major morbidity and mortality, respectively.[7] Although no studies to date have been carried out in patients with foregut disease alone, patients with serious mental illness are at increased risk for cardiovascular, respiratory, and gastrointestinal illnesses and carry higher rates of morbidity and mortality after general surgical intervention.[8,9]

The case of AH highlights the added complexity in diagnosis and initial management of upper gastrointestinal dysfunction in patients with mental illness. The underlying cognitive impairment of AH resulted in a social arrangement (an assisted-living facility with stakeholders other than her or her direct next-of-kin) that contributed to considerable delay in diagnosis. Prescribed use of PPIs indicates that she was previously evaluated for GERD; however, it was the accidental fall that caused her caretakers to seek medical attention and the bloody oral secretions suspected to be a result of lung or airway injury or secondary infection. Identification of rib fractures and lack of continued symptoms during the observation period in conjunction with her living situation may have misled providers from an acute work-up for hematemesis, otherwise considered an alarm finding. In retrospect, it is again clear that she continued to have symptoms because of GERD exacerbated by the presence of the hiatal hernia on each ensuing evaluation. Yet it was her behavioral decline that led to hospital admission for psychiatric treatment with her foregut disease remaining secondary up to the point of surgical emergency. Adjusted for other variables, inpatients with serious mental illness may undergo fewer operations than their peers.[9] Contributing factors to higher rates of morbidity and mortality in the seriously mentally ill patient in the outpatient setting include missed medical or surgical diagnoses, poor compliance or medication nonadherence, and treatment refusal.[10]

Although SS presented in extremis, and although an opportunity for nonelective intervention was not available, staging of her surgical approach was possible. Respect of metabolic status and resuscitation end points, and image reassessment are fundamental in establishing an effective operative approach. It is not uncommon for practitioners to hold a narrow, organ system–focused approach in their discussion with these patients and their families such that communication of the overall status of the patient, convalescence period, new limitations after convalescence including an increased level of care in the long term, medical costs, and long-term rehabilitation fails to occur. Information on habits, behaviors, language capacity and ability to follow medical advice, medications not on record, actual mobility and ambulation status before the acute process, diet preferences, sleep behavior, and potentially avoidable triggers of environmental stress play a greater role in establishing a plan of care for these patients. Failure to appreciate the legitimate baseline functional status and limitations of the patient has as severe an impact as lack of recognition of any technical aspect, with clear communication regarding all psychosocial factors bearing heavy influence on the understanding of the disease process and management of expectations of family and caretakers. With the assistance of an independent palliative care service when available, we place emphasis on such detailed discussions with family members and caregivers.

Recognizing the high morbidity and mortality of gangrenous stomach in the elderly and mentally ill, acutely decompensated patient, it is our practice to first perform endoscopic evaluation with an alpha loop maneuver to attempt decompression and detorsion.[11] Initial improvement in medical status with early metabolic correction over 48 to 72 hours allows for reimaging, cardiopulmonary evaluation, and assessment of any other pathology that may impact care and decision making before undertaking staged definitive intervention. We perform laparoscopic inspection and repair without the use of mesh in most cases, maintaining the principles to restore anatomy, high esophageal mediastinal mobilization, complete sac dissection with resection of nonviable tissue, vagal nerve and crural lining preservation, and tension-free crural repair.[12] Spine deformities, contractions, and abdominal chest anatomy may be altered and such maneuvers as instillation of a controlled CO_2 pneumothorax, splenophrenic attachments release, and lateral diaphragm release may be used to achieve tension-free closure.[13] Furthermore, this frequently bedridden population has an increased rate of cervical dysphagia, dysmotility, poor airway protection skills, and may have poor supervision at care centers. Therefore, accounting for an inordinately high risk of aspiration must play a part in the surgical strategy. Excessive pull on the stomach to compensate for insufficient intra-abdominal esophageal distance compromises the GEJ angle, creates a widely incompetent Hill valve, and imparts a high burden reflux. We perform gastropexy to the left hemidiaphragm while maintaining a GEJ angle and obtaining appropriate intra-abdominal esophagus length for these patients.[14] Medication regimens for baseline mental conditions must also be considered, because these frequently slow bowel transit. Frequently the pharmacodynamics and posology of these treatments have a limited menu, nonetheless liquid or crushable options are preferred to allow easier and safer passage. To limit the consequences of gastrointestinal bloating, pill retention and esophageal or Collis segment ulceration, which may be worsened by fundoplication, high esophageal mobilization for an appropriate intra-abdominal segment with an optimal crural repair, and gastric fundic fixation to a relaxed diaphragm is favored. The use of a gastrostomy tube for gastropexy, rather than feeding access alone, serves as a beneficial adjunct. This access allows for gastric venting in cases of vagal injury, transiently paretic stomach, and bloating medical regimens. Careful attention to abdominal esophageal length and GEJ angle must be observed. The stomach must lay in the abdomen of its own accord and a consequence of appropriately high esophageal mobilization. The gastrostomy is not a hook to hang the stomach under tension to fix its subdiaphragmatic location. Recurrent symptomatic proximal gastric herniations in the presence of G-tubes in the antrum are a cocktail for aspiration complications. Consideration of a jejunal access or extension limb off the G-tube is an option to palliate. Postoperative care follows the same principles as those used in standard patient populations, including early involvement of physical therapy, pulmonary therapy, and nutritional staff. Additional weight is given to speech and swallowing function evaluations before starting diets that add to the risk of aspiration, and nasogastric tubes may be kept longer than usual if oral route medication requirements are present.

THORACIC MALIGNANCY

Case 4

LR is a 68-year-old man with a past medical history significant for bipolar disorder and Asperger syndrome referred to our thoracic surgery practice after inpatient work-up and treatment of pneumonia identified a complex left lower lobe mass. He underwent bronchoscopy with endobronchial biopsy positive for adenocarcinoma, which crossed the fissure, requiring left thoracoscopic pneumonectomy and adjuvant chemotherapy (**Figs. 7** and **8**, Video 6). His postoperative course was significant for dysphagia requiring patient and family education and administration of antipsychotic medications, but he was otherwise able to convalesce and return home with family members.

Discussion

Surgical patients with serious mental illness have been shown to have worse clinical outcomes in comparison with those without, such that additional close attention to perioperative care is

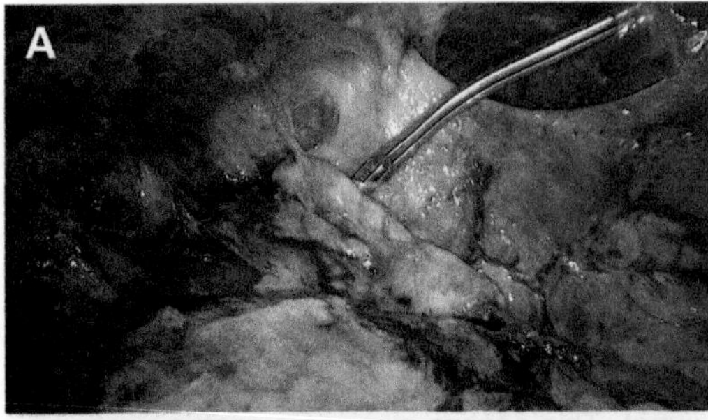

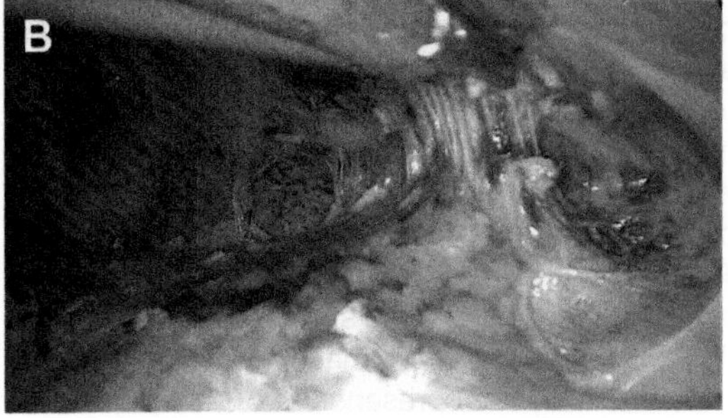

Fig. 7. (*A, B*) Postinduction therapy adhesions.

warranted.[8] Systemic effects of mental illness, including autonomic and thermoregulatory dysfunction, and the impact of medication management during the perioperative period may lead to higher rates of physiologic compromise.[8,15] Wherever possible, all aspects of oncologic care, physiologic management, anesthesia use, and postoperative considerations and disposition are planned in advance and communicated clearly and extensively with family and caregivers. As in other thoracic oncology patient populations, multispecialty discussion that may include psychiatry and palliative medicine is beneficial to follow sound oncologic principles of resection and lymphadenectomy while maintaining careful consideration of quality of life and long-term life expectancy. Traditional pulmonary function testing may not be feasible in cognitively limited states or presence of motor limitations. Partial volumes testing, body plethysmography, arterial blood gas analysis, 6-minute-walk oximetry, overnight oximetry, tilt bed cardiopulmonary testing, and ventilation perfusion scanning are some of the other aids for surgical plan. In some cases, parenchymal sparing and nonsurgical therapies, such as ablation and highly modulated forms of radiotherapy, may be most appropriate. Preoperative assessment of chest and spine deformities in this population allows for an improved intraoperative approach, because attention to detail prevents unnecessary accessory ports or open conversion in patients where minimal chest wall musculature compromise is of extreme importance. Port placements frequently require moving anteriorly in convex spines toward the side of disease or posteriorly on concave ones with increased anterior-posterior diameter. Spine curvature may limit the effective instrument work volumes and limit the thoracoscopic fulcrum effect. To preclude splinting in patients incapable of using demand dose systems, such as patient-controlled analgesia pumps in the postoperative period, we perform intraoperative rib blocks with long-lasting agents (Marcaine), use nonnarcotic topical patches, and provide scheduled narcotic pain management dosing along with more frequent nursing evaluations of mental status.

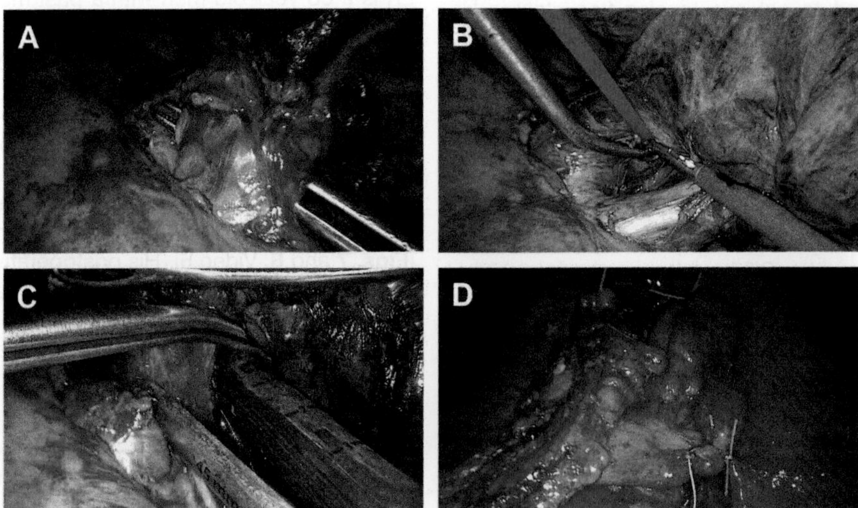

Fig. 8. Left thoracoscopic pneumonectomy. (*A*) Left superior pulmonary vein. (*B*) Left main pulmonary artery. (*C*) Left mainstem bronchus. (*D*) Vascularized pericardial fat patch.

SUMMARY

Optimized treatment of special care patients impels the thoracic surgery treatment team to recognize and act on additional considerations within each of the three phases of care. In the preoperative phase, attention should be directed toward cultivating a clear understanding of the goals of care and fostering shared, realistic outcomes of surgical intervention. Through the process of informed consent in the United States, surgeons have explicit ethical and legal obligations based on the standards of professional community and reasonable person, including, but not limited to, offering disclosure of all relevant details including the diagnosis, risks, benefits, expected outcomes, and treatment alternatives to the proposed procedure.[16] Although the mechanics can be cumbersome, the practice of consent is best viewed as an indelible vehicle for the development of a professional alliance, using bidirectional communication to establish goals of care and expectations in treatment.[16] Patients (or when appropriate, their surrogates) must assimilate clinical information, demonstrate understanding, and carry out their own process of decision making to include all information and influences.[16] Inconsistently emphasized in the clinical setting, the onus of discerning decision-making capacity lies with the surgeon.[17] Capacity is not infrequently overestimated among the elderly, those with subclinical mental illness, and those with neurodegenerative disease.[17] For the special care patient, this process should be approached thoughtfully and deliberately using screening tests for cognitive impairment, such as the Mini-Mental Status Examination or Clock Drawing Test, which can be performed and documented rapidly and easily by a member of the treatment team in either the outpatient or inpatient setting.

With a relative frequency of incurable disease and high incidence of patients with poor functional status, the use of palliative approaches in thoracic surgery is in no way novel.[18] The benefits of early palliative care specialist consultation are tangible and widespread, and preoperative palliative assessment is invaluable in treating the special care patient because decision-making in this setting can give rise to interpersonal conflict among the care team, patient, surrogates, and family and complex postoperative disposition planning.[18,19] In addition to the strategies of early tracheostomy and enteral access discussed previously, palliative approaches may also include management of nonmalignant, noninfected chronic effusions with tunneled pleural catheters (PleurX, BD Biosciences, San Jose, CA) that are more easily managed in the patient's postacute care environment; however, the infectious risks of these may be disastrous if appropriate hygiene and care is not maintained. A thoracoscopic surgical decortication is preferred when the mental illness state may be aggravated by catheters at the skin surface.

In an era of increasingly protocolized surgery, preoperative decision-making must be tailored to the goals of care, acknowledging and not avoiding the functional debilities and physiologic limitations of this distinctive patient population. Improving outcomes for these patients relies on clear and consistent communication to garner the support of hospital stakeholders, family, and caregivers, to establish the foundation for much-needed flexibility required in the operating room, and to minimize the stress related to lack of information of acute and long-term postoperative care.

SUPPLEMENTARY DATA

Supplementary data related to this article can be found online at https://doi.org/10.1016/j.thorsurg.2017.08.007.

REFERENCES

1. Vos T, Barber RM, Bell B, et al. Global, regional, and national incidence, prevalence, and years lived with disability for 301 acute and chronic diseases and injuries in 188 countries, 1990–2013: a systematic analysis for the Global Burden of Disease Study 2013. Lancet 2015;386:743–800.
2. Laughlin D, Brown M. Improving surgical outcomes for people with dementia. Nurs Stand 2015;29(38):50–8.
3. Gray DM, Kushnir V, Kalra G, et al. Cameron lesions in patients with hiatal hernias: prevalence, presentation, and treatment outcome. Dis Esophagus 2015;28:448–52.
4. Maganty K, Smith RL. Cameron lesions: unusual cause of gastrointestinal bleeding and anemia. Digestion 2008;77:214–7.
5. Cameron AJ, Higgins JA. Linear gastric erosion. A lesion associated with large diaphragmatic hernia and chronic blood loss anemia. Gastroenterology 1986;91(2):338–42.
6. Duranceau A. Massive hiatal hernia: a review. Dis Esophagus 2016;29:350–66.
7. Tan V, Luketich JD, Winger DG, et al. Non-elective paraesophageal hernia repair portends worse outcomes in comparable patients: a propensity-adjusted analysis. J Gastrointest Surg 2016;21(1):137–45.
8. Copeland LA, Zeber JE, Pugh MJ, et al. Postoperative complications in the seriously mentally ill: a

systematic review of the literature. Ann Surg 2008; 248:31–8.
9. Copeland LA, Sako EY, Zeber JF, et al. Mortality after cardiac or vascular operations by preexisting serious mental illness status in the Veterans Health Administration. Gen Hosp Psychiatry 2014;36:502–8.
10. Brown S, Inskip H, Barraclough B. Causes of the excess mortality of schizophrenia. Br J Psychiatry 2000;177:212–7.
11. Tsang TK, Walker R, Yu DJ. Endoscopic reduction of gastric volvulus: the alpha-loop maneuver. Gastrointest Endosc 1995;42(3):244–8.
12. Luketich JD, Nason KS, Christie NA, et al. Outcomes after a decade of laparoscopic giant paraesophageal hernia repair. J Thorac Cardiovasc Surg 2010; 139(2):395.
13. Schuchert MJ, Adusumilli PS, Cook CC, et al. The impact of scoliosis among patients with giant paraesophageal hernia. J Gastrointest Surg 2011;15: 23–8.
14. Louie BE, Kapur S, Blitz M, et al. Length and pressure of the reconstructed lower esophageal sphincter is determined by both crural closure and Nissen fundoplication. J Gastrointest Surg 2013;17: 236–43.
15. Kudoh A. Perioperative management for chronic schizophrenic patients. Anesth Analg 2005;101: 1867–72.
16. Jones JW, McCullough LB, Richman BW. A comprehensive primer of surgical informed consent. Surg Clin North Am 2007;87:903–18.
17. Terranova C, Cardin F, Di Pietra L, et al. Ethical and medico-legal implications of capacity of patients in geriatric surgery. Med Sci Law 2013;53(3):166–71.
18. Nelems B. Palliative care principles for thoracic surgery. Thorac Surg Clin 2013;23:443–6.
19. Freeman RK, Arevalo G, Ascioti AJ, et al. An assessment of the frequency of palliative procedures in thoracic surgery. J Surg Educ 2017. [Epub ahead of print].

Management of Lung Cancer with Concomitant Cardiac Disease

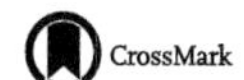

Benjamin Powell, MD[a], William D. Bolton, MD[b,*]

KEYWORDS

• Lung cancer • Heart disease • Coronary artery disease • Concomitant • Simultaneous

KEY POINTS

- Combined cardiac and thoracic surgery is an option for the subset of patients with synchronous cardiac and pulmonary surgical disease. Patients best suited for combined surgery are those with early-stage lung malignancy and cardiac disease not requiring emergent intervention.
- Performing lung resections while not on cardiopulmonary bypass is preferable due to bleeding concerns. No definitive evidence of metastatic risk of using bypass exists.
- One commonly cited drawback of oncologic pulmonary resections through a median sternotomy is inadequate or difficult mediastinal lymph node dissections, but no study has shown a significant difference.
- Although described over many years, this topic lacks level 1 evidence and most data are retrospective reviews of small patient series. Further evidence is needed on this topic.

INTRODUCTION: NATURE OF THE PROBLEM

It is common for patients presenting with a newly diagnosed lung mass to have concomitant cardiac disease. In the small number of patients who proceed to surgery for either cardiac or pulmonary disease, the standing question is, How is it best to treat these patients? For instance, should they have complete treatment of their cardiac disease followed by delayed resection of their lung cancer? Should they undergo other interventions, such as percutaneous coronary intervention (PCI), with angioplasty or stenting? Should they be offered surgery on both their heart and lungs under the same anesthesia? Should they undergo a sternotomy or a thoracotomy? Should the procedure utilize cardiopulmonary bypass (CPB) or be an off-pump procedure? Are short-term and long-term survival rates impacted? In a fairly complicated subject with a large amount of patient and disease variability, there are no well-established answers to these questions.

A variety of answers have evolved over time, but these are based on few data. In fact, few randomized or prospective trials have been published on this issue. To date, the largest study includes 79 patients, with the majority of studies ranging between 2 and 5 patients per year. There are 2 review articles in the literature, with the most recent published in 2014.[1,2] This article discusses the numerous issues surrounding lung cancer treatment in patients with concomitant cardiac disease. It addresses the preoperative work-up of these patients and the specifics of surgical intervention.

Disclosure: The authors have no commercial or financial conflicts to disclose.

[a] Department of Surgery, Greenville Health System, 701 Grove Road, 3rd Floor Support Tower, Greenville, SC 29605, USA; [b] Department of Surgery, Division of Thoracic Surgery, University of South Carolina, School of Medicine Greenville, 890 West Faris Road, Suite 320, Greenville, SC 29605, USA
* Corresponding author.
E-mail address: wbolton@ghs.org

Thorac Surg Clin 28 (2018) 69–79
https://doi.org/10.1016/j.thorsurg.2017.08.008

PATIENT POPULATION AND PRESENTATION

The Society of Thoracic Surgeons (STS) database reports a 20.9% incidence rate of coronary artery disease (CAD) in patients undergoing pulmonary resection for primary lung cancer.[3] These 2 conditions have multiple coinciding risk factors, including increased age, tobacco use, and lifestyle. As a result, a high overlap of patients with concomitant disease is expected. Despite the sizable incidence of concomitant disease, only 0.4% of coronary artery bypass grafts (CABGs) are combined procedures.[4]

Although some investigators argue that cardiac disease is not a significant risk factor for lung cancer resections, most agree it plays a significant role in patient outcomes. In 2008, Mishra and colleagues[5] examined more than 1000 patients and found no differences in morbidity or mortality in those with or without cardiac comorbidities. The investigators reported an overall myocardial infarction (MI) rate of 0.3% to 0.5% during the postoperative period.

The discovery of concomitant cardiac and pulmonary disease can occur simultaneously or one may be found in the preoperative work-up of the other. Most investigators report that it is more common for a lung mass to be found in work-up of cardiac disease than vice versa.[6–9] A Mayo clinic series done between 1965 and 1992 on 28,000 patients who underwent CABG identified 30 patients who had combined cardiac and pulmonary procedures via median sternotomy. From these 30 patients, 93% (n = 28) presented with cardiac symptoms and were found to have a pulmonary lesion on preoperative imaging. The remaining 2 patients (7%) presented with pulmonary symptoms.[10] Another US study involving a multicenter review of 3364 patients undergoing CABG identified 191 patients (5.7%) with pulmonary lesions preoperatively; a majority of these were benign. They reported a prevalence of 0.4% of pulmonary malignancy in patients undergoing CABG.[11]

Although a majority of studies have shown cardiac symptoms the more common initial complaint, several studies that looked solely at patients with concomitant cardiac disease and lung cancer have found a higher incidence of pulmonary complaints at presentation.[12,13] One possible reason for these findings may be explained by the fact that the patients in these studies were first seen in thoracic surgery clinics instead of an emergency room or cardiac surgery office; therefore, they were expected to have predominantly pulmonary symptoms at initial presentation.[12]

PREOPERATIVE ASSESSMENT

Diagnosis of both pulmonary and cardiac disease has evolved over the past several decades and now includes new modalities. One of these modalities is low-dose screening CT scan (LDCT), which is used for the detection of pulmonary nodules. Utilization of screening CT scans has increased significantly since Medicare approved coverage of LDCT for lung cancer in certain at-risk populations. The increased number of screening LDCTs led Mets and colleagues[14] from the Netherlands to create a model using screening CT scans to find lung cancers earlier and predict a patient's risk of cardiovascular disease. They used the same LDCTs to measure the coronary and aortic calcium volumes combined with demographic information to predict risk of cardiovascular events. Their validated model showed high-risk patients to have a 6% 3-year risk of having a cardiovascular event. As a result, they proposed that high-risk patients may benefit from preventative strategies, such as intense smoking cessation counseling.

Once a lung nodule has been found, a diagnosis should be obtained. This can be done with a percutaneous biopsy or endobronchial biopsy or at the time of resection. If possible, however, every effort should be taken to obtain the diagnosis preoperatively. After a diagnosis that warrants resection has been obtained, a preoperative risk assessment for their pulmonary and cardiac status is required.

From a cardiac standpoint most pulmonary resections are classified as an intermediate-risk or high-risk procedure, with 1% to 5% or greater than 5% chance of perioperative cardiac event, respectively.[15] The preoperative evaluation begins with a history and physical to elucidate symptoms of unstable coronary syndromes; these include MI within the past 30 days, decompensated heart failure, arrhythmias, or severe valvular disease.[16] If symptoms are discovered, then an evaluation by a cardiologist is recommended. This evaluation typically includes cardiac stress tests, heart catheterization, and, likely, intervention by cardiology for stabilization.

Based on 2014 American College of Cardiology/American Heart Association guidelines, indications for preoperative coronary revascularization prior to noncardiac surgery include significant left main disease, 3-vessel disease, and 2-vessel disease with left anterior descending stenosis with ejection fraction less than 50%. Revascularization can be performed with either PCI or CABG depending on the clinical scenario. If PCI is chosen, balloon angioplasty with a bare metal stent (BMS) placement over drug-eluting stent (DES) is preferable so that dual antiplatelet therapy (DAPT) can be held after 30 days instead of 6 months for a DES.[15]

Preoperative evaluation of the patient's pulmonary status begins with pulmonary function tests. Depending on the adequacy of these results, additional and more invasive pulmonary evaluation may be indicated. Judgment should be used, however, prior to obtaining a maximum oxygen consumption test (Vo_{2max}) due to the cardiac risk that can be encountered with the test itself. Patients with pulmonary reserve so marginal to require a Vo_{2max} study to determine if resection is possible may be best served with other treatment options for their lung malignancy, such as radiation or ablation therapy.

Patients with concomitant cardiac disease and lung cancer more frequently require a stabilizing intervention prior to pulmonary resection. Some patients, however, with poor pulmonary or cardiac status, may not be able to tolerate a procedure for either disease.

THERAPEUTIC OPTIONS AND/OR SURGICAL TECHNIQUE

When combined cardiac disease and lung cancer are encountered, there are 3 options for management: (1) PCI followed by treatment of the cancer, (2) combined cardiac and pulmonary operations, and (3) staged operative procedures.

Percutaneous Coronary Intervention

In 1994, Thomas and colleagues[17] published one of the first studies to explore PCI for patients with lung cancer undergoing resection. Between 1987 and 1992, they reviewed 21 patients with resectable non–small cell lung cancer (NSCLC) and CAD evident on a preoperative heart catheterization. Three of these patients had preoperative CABG, 4 had PCI with stenting, 2 were excluded due to poor cardiac function, and the remaining 12 patients had pulmonary resection without cardiac intervention. Mean delay to lung cancer resection was 41 days and postoperative mortality was 5.3%. There were more cardiac complications in the group that did not receive preoperative cardiac intervention. Based on these results, the investigators advocated staged coronary revascularization prior to lung resection.[17]

In 2002, Ciriaco and colleagues[12] examined how their department addressed CAD prior to pulmonary resection in 50 patients with lung cancer. Six patients had a preoperative CABG, 13 had a coronary angioplasty with 6 receiving a stent, and 31 had no intervention. There were no significant differences in postoperative complications among the groups who received preoperative CABG, PCI, or no intervention. Two deaths in the group with no preoperative intervention were medium-risk to high-risk patients with negative heart catheterizations. Intervention on cardiac disease prior to pulmonary resection was not found predictive of postoperative complications, whereas age and preoperative cardiac risk were.

In 2006, Brichon and colleagues[18] looked at BMS thrombosis after different durations of DAPT after stent placement and prior to lung resection. There were 32 patients who received a BMS followed by surgical resection with variable periods of DAPT (<30 days, n = 7; 30–60 days, n = 17; and 61–90 days, n = 8). There were 3 in-stent thromboses in this study, 2 of which occurred in the 30-day DAPT group. The other occurred 44 days post-PCI and led to reinfarction and death. Although this study is small, they found an in-stent thrombosis rate of 9%, which is significantly higher than the expected thrombosis rate (<1%) found in those who do not require discontinuation of their DAPT. They concluded that patients undergoing PCI before lung resection should have coronary angioplasty instead of stenting or should have DAPT continued perioperatively.

More recently in 2013, Fernandez and colleagues[19] looked at Medicare data of more than 22,000 patients undergoing pulmonary resection for lung cancer. They found that patients who underwent PCI with stenting within 12 months prior to surgery had a statistically significant increase in 30-day cardiac events (9.3%) and mortality (7.7%) compared with the group without prior stenting (4.9% and 4.6%). The investigators also reported a 10-fold increase in perioperative in-stent thrombosis or MI in the stent group compared with the no-stent group (3.1% vs 0.32%). DES was not included in their analysis because it was not widely used during that time period. After controlling for several variables, patients who had a stent placed in the preceding 12 months were associated with a 50% increased risk of operative mortality than those without a stent.

Staged Versus Combined Procedures

Historically, the preferred method for the treatment of patients with both operable cardiac and pulmonary disease was a staged procedure. The cardiac procedure was typically performed first, followed by the pulmonary resection once the patient had recovered from the cardiac operation. This recovery period is usually between 2 weeks and 8 weeks. Performance of staged procedures avoids issues, such as longer duration of the procedure, use of CPB with heparinization during the lung resection, and resection performed through a median sternotomy. This staged approach, however, requires patients to undergo 2 major operations and wait to have their lung cancer resected, potentially allowing for progression of disease.

When deciding if a patient is at an increased risk from a staged or combined approach, patient's associated risk with an isolated procedure must first be determined. Risks associated with lung resection have been well established. A single-center review of 634 lung resections from 1990 to 1997 showed an overall mortality rate of 3.2% and a major complication rate of 2.1%. Mortality for lobectomy alone was 1.2%. There were 10 cardiovascular complications, including 5 MIs. They identified independent risk factors for mortality; these included a history of CAD, pneumonectomy, and an increased American Society of Anesthesiology (ASA) classification.[20]

A larger study based on the STS database, in 2010, found a mortality rate of 2.2% for an isolated lung resection for primary lung cancer and a major morbidity rate of 6.4%.[4] Predictors of mortality in this study included pneumonectomy, bilobectomy, ASA classification, renal disease, use of neoadjuvant chemoradiation, steroid usage, age, urgent procedure, male gender, decreased forced expiratory volume in the first second of expiration, and body mass index (BMI). Risks associated with cardiac surgery are also well established. A study by Chung and colleagues[21] in 2015 using the American College of Surgeons National Surgical Quality Improvement Program database found an average mortality rate for an isolated CABG to be 2.2%. Predictors of mortality for this procedure are similar to those found for lung resections and include renal disease, age, and poor pulmonary function.

To date, studies on staged versus combined operations provide the best data on risks associated with undergoing both cardiac and pulmonary procedures. These studies identified a large number of variables in combined procedures, including patient factors, comorbidities, type of cardiac or lung procedure, utilization of a sternotomy or thoracotomy, use of CPB, and cancer type and stage. Most studies have controlled for patient factors and comorbidities. Median sternotomy was the most common approach for both procedures. There was significant variability in the use of CPB (on-pump vs off-pump) and the timing of lung resection in relation to the use of CPB (before-pump vs after-pump). On review of the literature, the most common reported cardiac procedure was CABG. Most of the lung cancers were T1 or T2 and N0 or N1.[2]

The earliest publications of combined cardiac and pulmonary procedures, aside from those for congenital malformations or iatrogenic injuries, include a few small case series.[22–24]

Rosalion and colleagues[25] looked at 10 patients with combined procedures and found 1 perioperative (10%) death from sepsis and 3 deaths within 13 months from recurrent cancer. Based on their experience, "early morbidity is mainly related to the cardiac procedure and impaired respiratory function preoperatively, but the long-term results are dependent upon on the control of the lung carcinoma."

In 1995, the Texas Heart Institute published their 18-year experience (1973–1990) with concomitant procedures totaling 21 patients. The procedures were predominantly CABGs with lobectomy; however, there were several valve replacement surgeries. They performed the lung resection at all points during the procedure: before CPB, on CPB but before the cardiac procedure, on CPB but after the cardiac procedure, and after CPB. They reported a 5-year survival of 52% with 1 perioperative death (5%) due to MI. No differences in bleeding or reoperation rate were seen in the use of CPB. The investigators concluded that concomitant surgery was safe and prevented patients from having a second major operation.[26]

In 1996, Johnson and colleagues[11] reviewed 3364 consecutive patients who underwent CABG, from which 191 patients (5%) had a lung nodule found on preoperative chest radiograph. From these, 151 had a granuloma. Of the remaining 40 patients, 18 underwent a combined cardiac procedure and resection of lung nodule via median sternotomy. A total of 15 patients (of 40) had a tissue diagnosis of malignancy, including 3 nodules that were not resected at the time of CABG but were followed with imaging and resected at a later time. Johnson and colleagues[11] reported a mortality rate of 5.5% for combined procedures compared with their reported rate of 3% for CABGs alone. Based on these data, the investigators recommend combined procedures when a preoperative diagnoses is attained or when the lesion is high risk.

In 1997, Voets and colleagues[27] performed a single-center review to compare combined procedures in 24 patients versus staged procedures in 10 patients. They focused on early-stage lung cancer (stages I or II). Median survival was 4.2 years and was comparable between groups. They reported a difference in perioperative mortality with 5 (20%) deaths in the combined procedure group versus 1 (10%) death in the staged group; this difference, however, was not statistically significant. In the staged group, the second operation (lung resection) occurred an average of 34 days after the cardiac operation. Time between procedures was not shown to influence mortality. Late deaths were attributable to recurrent or metastatic lung cancer.

One of the most cited series comparing staged to combined operations came from the Mayo Clinic. They looked 2604 CABGs and found 30 patients who underwent combined operations compared with 15 patients who underwent staged operations between 1965 and 1992. Both groups included mixed cardiac and pulmonary procedures. The 5-year survival was 35% in the combined group and 53% in the staged group. Of patients with stage I disease, the 5-year survival was 37% in the combined group and 100% in the staged group. The perioperative mortality rate for the combined group was 6.7%, compared with 0% for the staged group. They concluded that patients should not undergo simultaneous operations unless they can tolerate a second procedure.[10]

Operative Approach

Sternotomy versus thoracotomy

Most cardiac procedures are traditionally carried out through a median sternotomy for exposure to the heart and other mediastinal structures. Lung resections have traditionally been performed through thoracotomies. There was a period of time in the 1970s and 1980s in which multiple articles were published advocating for median sternotomy as a standard approach for lung resections. Some studies reported decreased postoperative pain, shorter hospital stays,[28] decreased pain medication usage,[29] and faster recovery[30] in the sternotomy group compared with thoracotomies. Investigators noted specific indications for sternotomy, such as bilateral pulmonary lesions.[31]

Asaph and colleagues[32] reported their long-term experience (1980–1994) using median sternotomy for resection of primary lung cancer. These data were obtained using a prospectively maintained database. They had 447 sternotomy patients and 368 thoracotomy patients. Right-sided, bilateral, and upper lobe lesions were approached more frequently by sternotomy. Postoperative bleeding was more common in the sternotomy group, but hospital stay was shorter by 24 hours. There was no significant difference in 5-year or 10-year survival between the 2 groups. There was a 0.9% incidence of deep sternal wound infections after sternotomy compared with a 2.2% rate of infection in their thoracotomy incisions. The perioperative mortality rate was 3.8% for the sternotomy group and 3.3% for the thoracotomy group.

There are several case reports of other operative approaches for combined surgery. Ahmed and colleagues[33] published a case report of a 61-year-old man who had an off-pump CABG combined with a left upper lobectomy through a left posterolateral thoracotomy. He had symptomatic coronary disease with a history of 2 previous MIs. On heart catheterization, his dominant coronary lesion was of the marginal circumflex artery. His preoperative work-up revealed a left upper lobe carcinoma. The lobectomy was performed first, followed by an off-pump saphenous vein graft.

A second case report by Mitropoulos and colleagues[34] noted use of a specialized T-bar retractor for exposure of the left internal mammary artery for a CABG combined with a left upper lobectomy with full lymph node dissection. The article points out that some situations are more advantageous for combined procedures. They indicate, as is commonly noted, that a median sternotomy offers adequate exposure for left upper lobectomies but poor exposure for left lower lobectomies. In some cases, revascularizing the myocardium first may be safer; however, this places the left internal mammary artery graft at risk of damage during the lung resection.

Multiple investigators note that the mediastinal lymph node dissection, particularly more posteriorly, is more difficult through a median sternotomy compared with a posterolateral thoracotomy.[1,4,6,13,35–37] Miller and colleagues[10] noted a difference in 5-year survival between their combined (35%) and staged (53%) operations. In patients with stage I disease, the 5-year survival was 37% in the combined group and 100% in the staged group. They attributed this to understaging of disease in the combined group likely due to poor lymph node dissections via median sternotomy. Pathology revealed N2 disease in only 3% of patients in the combined group versus 33% in the staged group (p<.01). These are some of the most compelling data supporting the opinion that median sternotomy yields an inferior lymph node dissection compared with a dedicated thoracic procedure. To date, there are not adequate data to comment on the adequacy of mediastinal lymph node dissections via a median sternotomy. If the approach of sternotomy contributes to staging bias, other preoperative or intraoperative methods, such as mediastinoscopy and endobronchial ultrasound, should be used for biopsy and staging of the mediastinum.

Exposure for the left upper lobectomies is more easily completed via a median sternotomy than other lobar resections, specifically a left lower lobectomy. Many investigators note that a left lower lobectomy is more difficult to complete by a median sternotomy due to the heart impeding the exposure to the inferior pulmonary ligament and nodal station.[1,7,8,30,35] When approaching the pleural spaces through a median sternotomy, increased attention should be paid to the course of the phrenic nerves when entering the pleural space because they may not be as well visualized from the medial position. Use of stay sutures in the pericardium as well as gauze or laparotomy pads placed behind the lung can be helpful to bring the hilum up into the operative field. The internal mammary arteries must be protected if they are to be grafted or have already been grafted at the time of the pulmonary operation. The addition of a camera though a port in the chest wall can also facilitate better visualization of the more lateral or posterior structures. Patients undergoing combined cardiac and pulmonary procedures who require an anterior chest wall resection may be best served by a thoracotomy.[1,9]

The question of adequacy of median sternotomy for resection of a primary lung lesion may not be as relevant as it previously was with the increased use of minimally invasive techniques both in cardiac and lung surgeries. Video-assisted thoracic surgery and robotic-assisted lung resections have become commonplace. Minimally invasive valve placements with minithoracotomies or by endovascular approaches have also increased in prevalence. Fewer procedures are requiring the exposure of a median sternotomy or thoracotomy. Lu and colleagues[38] presented a case of a patient who underwent a combined triple-vessel CABG and a left upper lobectomy with lymph node dissection. This was performed through a left parasternal minithoracotomy and use of a thoracoscope to assist in pulmonary and lymph node dissection.

On-Pump Versus Off-Pump

One of the most thoroughly studied topics in combined cardiac and pulmonary surgeries is the use of CPB. The negative effects of CPB have been well established and include increased bleeding risk from heparinization, tissue edema, and immunosuppression in the setting of cancer.[1,7,8,13,36,37,39,40] CPB is believed to cause immunosuppression by complement activation and interference with natural killer cell, T-cell, and neutrophil function.[1] In regard to cancer patients, there is the theoretic possibility of increasing the incidence of metastatic disease.[1,27] CABGs and other cardiac procedures can be performed with CPB (on-pump), or without CPB (off-pump). Bleeding associated with CPB can be related to multiple factors; these include overheparinization, inadequate heparin reversal, overdosing of protamine, and platelet dysfunction secondary to the extracorporeal circuit.[1] Combined procedures may also increase the need for blood transfusions, causing further immunosuppression. If CPB is necessary and is going to be used, the pulmonary resection and lymph node dissection can be performed prior to, during, or after CPB and the cardiac procedure. The best literature on this topic is reviewed.

With Cardiopulmonary Bypass (On-Pump)

One of the earliest studies on this topic is from Piehler and colleagues[6] who described 43 patients who had combined cardiac operations and lung resection between 1965 and 1983. A majority of the pulmonary lesions (93%) were found during preoperative cardiac work-up. Only 2 patients had a preoperative pulmonary diagnosis. Twelve patients were found to have a malignancy, 10 of which were primary lung cancer. From the 10 lung cancer patients, 6 patients had a lobectomy, 3 had a wedge resection, and 1 had a pneumonectomy. Most resections were performed after CPB (n = 21) compared with 6 during bypass and 16 prior to initiating bypass. There was 1 patient (2.3%) taken back for bleeding. They reported 2 perioperative deaths (4.6%), 1 of which was secondary to respiratory failure after the patient underwent resection of a metastasis from the wall of the right ventricle with 7 separate wedge resections for metastatic renal cell carcinoma and developed significant intrapulmonary bleeding while anticoagulated on bypass. The investigators concluded that lung resections are safely performed in concomitant surgery while off CPB.

Ulicny and colleagues[36] reported 19 patients who underwent combined procedures evaluating the impact of CPB on morbidity, perioperative mortality, and long-term survival. Fifteen (79%) patients had their resection while on CPB, 2 patients (11%) after CPB, and 3 (11%) before CPB. Bleeding complications were seen in 16% (n = 3) of patients. One patient developed bleeding after heparinization from a wedge staple line performed before CPB and required a completion lobectomy. Another patient required reoperation for bleeding from a staple line of a wedge resection performed while on CPB. There was 1 postoperative death (5%) due to adult respiratory distress syndrome after intraoperative bleeding complications after CPB and reversal. Survival of patients with stage I or stage II disease was 60% at 5 years and was not influenced by resection on CPB, type of resection, or postoperative complications. The investigators concluded that pulmonary resections should not be performed on CPB and staged procedures should be performed if possible.

In the largest series to date, Brutel de la Riviere and colleagues[9] presented their experience with 79 patients from 1979 to 1993. Their patients most commonly had stage I disease (66%), had squamous cell cancer (61%), and received a lobectomy (76%). No wedge resections were performed. All patients had a sternotomy and 11 patients had a thoracotomy in addition to the sternotomy. The first 10 patients in the series were operated on using intermittent aortic cross-clamping and hypothermia. In the patients who had a sternotomy alone, 33 had their pulmonary procedures before CPB, 27 during, and 8 after bypass; 5 while off bypass but still heparinized; and 3 after protamine. A total of 7 patients (9%) returned to the operating room for bleeding complications. The investigators noted an improved survival in the patients who had lung resection prior to CPB compared with those who had their resection during CPB, although this was not statistically significant. The overall in-hospital mortality rate was 6.3%. Patients who had sternotomy alone compared with sternotomy with a thoracotomy had a significantly improved perioperative mortality rate (2.9% vs 27.2%) and long-term survival rate (5.8 years vs 2.8 years). One patient (5%) had a phrenic nerve injury and palsy. Two-year and 5-year survival rates were 62% and 42%, respectively. Patients who underwent lung resection prior to CPB had a significantly improved survival rate compared with resection while on CPB (4.6 vs 3.8 years, respectively). More cardiac deaths were seen in the patients resected during CPB. Lung cancer accounted for 64% of late deaths.

A follow-up by Brutel de la Riviere and colleagues evaluated 43 patients who underwent combined procedures between 1994 and 2005. Lung resection was performed before CPB in 28 patients and 15 procedures were done off-pump. The CPB group had 1 bleeding complication (4%) and 4 infectious complications (14%) leading to 3 deaths (11%). Two-year and 5-year survival rates were statistically higher in the CPB group compared with the off-pump group, 58% versus 47% and 35% versus 13%, respectively. The off-pump group was older and had more advanced-stage lung malignancy. Long-term survival was improved in patients without recurrent CAD who had stage I cancer. They concluded that patient outcomes in combined procedures was not significantly different, regardless of whether the procedures was done on-pump or off-pump.[7]

Cathenis and colleagues[8] presented 27 patients who received a combined procedure between 2000 and 2008. Thirteen lung resections were done prior to CPB, 5 during, 3 after reversal of heparin, and 6 were off-pump. Bleeding complications were recorded in 3 patients (11%) requiring reoperation. CPB and timing of lung resection did not have an impact on long-term survival. Similar to other studies, the investigators showed the performance of a left lower lobectomy through a sternotomy while patients were on CPB to be easier than before or after CPB; this is likely due to the heart being able to be retracted more freely.[41]

In 1990, Canver and colleagues[42] reviewed 21 patients who underwent combined cardiac and pulmonary operations. Twelve patients had a pulmonary resection before CPB and 9 after bypass. There were no bleeding complications in either group. There was 1 perioperative death (5%) secondary to mediastinitis and sepsis. There was an overall 5-year survival of 88% in the 8 patients diagnosed with primary lung cancer. There was no significant difference in survival between the 2 groups.

In 1998, Danton and colleagues[1] reviewed 13 patients who had concomitant cardiac and pulmonary surgery. Two were performed without CPB, 1 after CPB due to emergent arrhythmia, and the remaining 10 prior to CPB. No bleeding complications and no perioperative mortality were reported. The investigators favored anatomic resections to decrease the chance of parenchymal bleeding. A difference in estimated blood loss was found between the off-pump group (average 300 mL) and the group who used CPB (926 mL).

In summary, patients undergoing a combined cardiac and pulmonary procedure with CPB seem to have significantly higher complication and mortality rates than expected from undergoing either procedure independently. It also seems from these studies that survival is more dependent on the stage of malignancy rather than the timing of the resection in regard to bypass. When looking at the bleeding risk for these combined procedures, if the resection is done with CPB, the reported bleeding rate is between 0 and 16%. The perioperative mortality rate is between 4.6% and 6.3% and the 5-year survival is 13% to 88%. The data on this topic have led many investigators to conclude that combined procedures are safe and can be advantageous for certain patients. The debate on this issue continues, because several investigators advocate for staged procedures.

Without Cardiopulmonary Bypass (Off-Pump)

Several investigators have advocated for combined pulmonary resection and off-pump cardiac surgery in patients requiring both procedures. Certainly this approach for patients with both cardiac and pulmonary disease is limited to cardiac procedures that are amenable to an off-pump approach. When looking at the studies investigating this topic, there are several common themes. Off-pump cardiac procedures seem able to be combined with pulmonary resections, because they have a low risk of bleeding (0%–8%) and perioperative mortality (0%) and have satisfactory long-term survival (55%–75%).[2,4,13,18,43]

Dyszkiewicz and colleagues[4] in 2004 presented 13 patients who had an off-pump CABG followed by lung resection. Patients received a mean of 1.7 grafts but were not candidates for endovascular intervention. Despite no heparinization, 1 patient (8%) required reoperation for bleeding. There were no perioperative mortalities in this study. The investigators recommend combining operations when the CABG can be done first, off-pump, and the patients only require 1 or 2 grafts.

A subsequent study by the same group evaluated 25 patients who had combined surgeries between 2001 and 2006. Twenty patients had a sternotomy and 4 had a left thoracotomy. All patients had an off-pump CABG prior to lung resection. One patient (4%) had a reoperation for bleeding and 1 patient (4%) developed a bronchopleural fistula. There were no perioperative deaths and the 3-year survival rate was 50%. The only factor shown to have an impact on long-term survival was cancer recurrence, which was seen in 55% of the patients in this study. Preoperatively they excluded patients with N2 disease; however, 2 patients were discovered to have N2 disease on final pathology and did well after receiving adjuvant treatment.[43]

Recently Ma and colleagues[13] published their 12-year experience with 34 patients undergoing an off-pump CABG and pulmonary resection. They excluded patients from analysis if the final pathology was not primary lung cancer. A greater number of their patients presented with pulmonary complaints than cardiac (65%). Early patients in their series had an off-pump CABG via median sternotomy, were repositioned, and then a lung resection via thoracotomy. Later they transitioned to performing lobectomies through the sternotomy with the assistance of a thoracoscope, predominantly for lymph node dissection.[18] Compared with their patients who received an off-pump CABG alone, the addition of a pulmonary resection did not increase their overall rate of complication (21%), which included respiratory complications and arrhythmias. There was no perioperative bleeding requiring reoperation or mortality. Three-year and 5-year survival rates were 75% and 67%, respectively.[13] Several other small case series found similar results to these larger studies.[37,40,44,45]

Table 1
Summary of primary outcomes for patients with concomitant cardiac disease and lung cancer undergoing surgery—combined procedures versus staged

	Combined Procedures (%)	Staged (%)
Reoperation for bleeding	0–11	0
Operative mortality	0–20.8	0–10
1-y survival	79–100	72.7
5-y survival	34.9–85	53

Data from Tourmousoglou C, Apostolakis E, Dougenis D. Simultaneous occurrence of coronary artery disease and lung cancer: what is the best surgical treatment strategy? Interact Cardiovasc Thorac Surg 2014;19:673–81.

In 2014, a review article for simultaneous coronary and lung cancer surgery was published by Tourmousoglou and colleagues[2] they used a best evidence protocol developed for cardiothoracic surgery and included 15 retrospective studies from 1994 to 2012. They tabulated the results of those studies for easy comparison and were able to report the ranges for all key outcomes (**Table 1**). Their review confirmed many of the same conclusions made by others. They determined that combined procedures can be safely performed in patients with stage I and stage II lung cancers; however, there are high-risk patients who likely would be better served by staged surgeries. Long-term survival is most dependent on the patients' cancer stage. They noted that off-pump CABG seemed a safe method for combined operations. They also found an aggregate mortality rate for off-pump combined operations of 0% to 6.6%. The risk of bleeding in these patients ranged from 0% to 4%, and 5-year survival ranged from 13% to 68%. Their data suggested that when CPB is used, the pulmonary resection should be performed first.

SUMMARY

Combined cardiac and pulmonary procedures are well described, although there are few evidence-based guidelines. Almost all of the published data on the topic are retrospective chart reviews.

Patients more often present with cardiac symptoms and are found to have pulmonary pathology on preoperative imaging. The vast majority of patients are men. There are 3 main options for patients with concomitant cardiac and pulmonary surgical processes: staged operations, PCI preoperatively, and combined operations of multiple varieties. Combined procedures via sternotomy are more beneficial in some patients, such as those undergoing bilateral lung procedures. Most pulmonary procedures can be performed via a median sternotomy. Certain lung resections, such as left lower lobectomy, may be more difficult to perform via a median sternotomy. Median sternotomy offers some benefits over traditional thoracotomy, including decreased postoperative pain, decreased length of stay, and reduced operative time. Relative contraindications to pulmonary resection via median sternotomy include chest wall involvement (T3 lesion), high bleeding risk, and extensive intrathoracic adhesions. Mediastinal lymph node dissection of certain lymph node stations, such as posterior paraesophageal and inferior pulmonary ligament nodes, may be more difficult when performed through a sternotomy. Most investigators agree combined procedures should be reserved for stage I and stage II NSCLC and not be performed with patients with N2 or T3 disease. Preoperative staging with imaging, mediastinoscopy, or other modality, such as endobronchial ultrasound-guided biopsy that was not previously available, is appropriate. There may be a higher bleeding risk for those lung resections performed while anticoagulated on CPB. The impact of the other immunologic effects of bypass on patients with lung cancer is not clearly defined. There is no clear evidence that CPB increases the risk of metastatic disease in patients with pulmonary malignancy. Off-pump CABG seems to have a decreased risk of bleeding and perioperative mortality compared with on-pump combined procedures, when reviewing the small studies in the literature. This may be related to improved results or reflect a bias in patient selection.

Average hospital length of stay for combined cardiac and pulmonary surgeries: 10 days to 20 days.[25,46] Average stay for lung cancer resection alone was 5 days. This topic is quickly changing with new minimally invasive techniques. Minimally invasive and endovascular techniques, such as transcatheter aortic valve replacement (TAVR), may continue to shorten hospital length of stay even further. There is 1 reported case of a combined transapical aortic valve replacement with a traditional lobectomy via thoracotomy[46] but none of thoracic procedures combined with TAVR. A recent editorial noted that many studies of TAVR note active neoplasm as a contraindication, excluding patients with thoracic oncologic pathology from being candidates for TAVR.[47] Combined procedures may offer fewer benefits in terms of postoperative pain levels, length of stay, and recovery times. Further study of this data may be an area for research in the future. A multicenter prospectively maintained database would be useful in a rare topic such as "combined cardiac procedures with concomitant pulmonary resection".

REFERENCES

1. Danton MH, Anikin VA, McManus KG, et al. Simultaneous cardiac surgery with pulmonary resection: presentation of series and review of literature. Eur J Cardiothorac Surg 1998;13:667–72.
2. Tourmousoglou C, Apostolakis E, Dougenis D. Simultaneous occurrence of coronary artery disease and lung cancer: what is the best surgical treatment strategy? Interact Cardiovasc Thorac Surg 2014;19:673–81.
3. Kozower BD, Sheng S, O'brien SM, et al. STS database risk models: predictors of mortality and major morbidity for lung cancer resection. Ann Thorac Surg 2010;90:875–83.
4. Dyszkiewicz W, Jemielity MM, Piwkowski CT, et al. Simultaneous lung resection for cancer and myocardial revascularization without cardiopulmonary bypass (off-pump coronary artery bypass grafting). Ann Thorac Surg 2004;77:1023–7.
5. Mishra PK, Pandey R, Michael J, et al. Cardiac comorbidity is not a risk factor for mortality and morbidity following surgery for primary non-small cell lung cancer. Eur J Cardiothorac Surg 2009;35:439–43.
6. Piehler JM, Trastek VF, Pairolero PC, et al. Concomitant cardiac and pulmonary operations. J Thorac Cardiovasc Surg 1985;90:662–7.
7. Schoenmakers MC, van Boven WJ, van den Bosch JV, et al. Comparison of on-pump or off-pump coronary artery revascularization with lung resection. Ann Thorac Surg 2007;84:504–9.
8. Cathenis K, Hamerlijnck R, Vermassen F, et al. Concomitant cardiac surgery and pulmonary resection. Acta Chir Belg 2009;109:306–11.
9. Brutel de la Riviere A, Knaepen P, Vanswieten H, et al. Concomitant open heart surgery and pulmonary resection for lung cancer. Eur J Cardiothorac Surg 1995;9:310–4.
10. Miller D, Orszulak T, Pairolero P, et al. Combined operation for lung cancer and cardiac disease. Ann Thorac Surg 1994;58:989–94.
11. Johnson J, Landreneau R, Boley T, et al. Should pulmonary lesions be resected at the time of open heart surgery? Amer Surg 1996;62:300–3.
12. Ciriaco P, Carretta A, Calori G, et al. Lung resection for cancer in patients with coronary arterial disease:

analysis of short-term results. Eur J Cardiothorac Surg 2002;22:35–40.
13. Ma X, Huang F, Zhang Z, et al. Lung cancer resection with concurrent off pump coronary artery bypasses: safety and efficiency. J Thorac Dis 2016;8:2038–45.
14. Mets OM, Vliegenthart R, Gondrie MJ, et al. Lung cancer screening CT-based prediction of cardiovascular events. JACC Cardiovasc Imaging 2013;6:899–907.
15. Levine GN, Bates ER, Bittl JA, et al. 2016 ACC/AHA guideline focused update on duration of dual antiplatelet therapy in patients with coronary artery disease: a report of the American College of Cardiology/American Heart Association task force on clinical practice guidelines. Circulation 2016;134:123–55.
16. Sugarbaker DJ, Bueno R, Colson YL, et al. Adult chest surgery. 2nd edition. New York: McGraw-Hill Education; 2015.
17. Thomas P, Giudicelli R, Guillen J, et al. Is lung cancer surgery justified in patients with coronary artery disease? Eur J Cardiothorac Surg 1994;8:287–92.
18. Brichon P, Boitet P, Dujon A, et al. Perioperative in-stent thrombosis after lung resection performed within 3 months of coronary stenting. Eur J Cardiothorac Surg 2006;30:793–6.
19. Fernandez FG, Crabtree TD, Liu J, et al. Incremental risk of prior coronary arterial stents for pulmonary resection. Ann Thorac Surg 2013;95:1212–20.
20. Licker M. Perioperative mortality and major cardiopulmonary complications after lung surgery for non-small cell carcinoma. Eur J Cardiothorac Surg 1999;15:314–9.
21. Chung PJ, Carter TI, Burack JH, et al. Predicting the risk of death following coronary artery bypass graft made simple: a retrospective study using the American college of surgeons national surgical quality improvement program database. J Cardiothorac Surg 2015;10:62.
22. Dalton ML, Parker TM, Mistrot JJ, et al. Concomitant coronary artery bypass and major noncardiac surgery. J Thorac Cardiovasc 1978;75:621–4.
23. Bricker DL, Parker DM, Dalton ML, et al. Open heart surgery with concomitant pulmonary resection. Cardiovasc Dis 1980;7:411–9.
24. Girardet RE, Masri ZH, Lansin AM. Pulmonary lesions in patients undergoing open heart surgery. Approach and management. J Ky Med Assoc 1981;79:645–8.
25. Rosalion A, Woodford NW, Clarke CP, et al. Concomitant coronary revascularization and resection of lung cancer. Aust N Z J Surg 1993;63:336–40.
26. La Francesca S, Frazier OH, Radovancěvić B, et al. Concomitant cardiac and pulmonary operations for lung cancer. Tex Heart Inst J 1995;22:296–300.
27. Voets A, Joesoef KS, van Teeffelen ME. Synchroneously occurring lung cancer (stages I–II) and coronary artery disease: concomitant versus staged surgical approach. Eur J Cardiothorac Surg 1997;12:713–7.
28. Urschel UC, Razzuk MA. Median sternotomy as a standard approach for pulmonary resection. Ann Thorac Surg 1986;41:130–4.
29. Asaph JW, Keppel JF. Midline sternotomy for the treatment of primary pulmonary neoplasms. Am J Surg 1984;147:589–92.
30. Cooper JD, Nelems JM, Pearson FG. Extended indications for median sternotomy in patients requiring pulmonary resection. Ann Thorac Surg 1978;26:413–20.
31. Meng RL, Jensik RJ, Kittle CF, et al. Median sternotomy for synchronous bilateral pulmonary operations. J Thorac Cardiovasc Surg 1980;80:1–7.
32. Asaph JW, Handy JR, Grunkemeier GL, et al. Median sternotomy versus thoracotomy to resect primary lung cancer: analysis of 815 cases. Ann Thorac Surg 2000;70:373–9.
33. Ahmed AA, Sarsam MA. Off-pump combined coronary artery bypass grafting and left upper lobectomy through left posterolateral thoracotomy. Ann Thorac Surg 2001;71:2016–8.
34. Mitropoulos F, Kanakis MA, Apostolou A, et al. T-bar utilization for concomitant coronary artery bypass graft operation and left upper lobectomy. Case Rep Surg 2016;2016:1–2.
35. Brutel de la Riviere A. Concomitant cardiac and pulmonary operations. 1st edition. General thoracic surgery, Vol 7. Philidelphia: Lippincott Williams & Wilkins; 2009. p. 537–40.
36. Ulicny KS, Schmelzer V, Flege JB, et al. Concomitant cardiac and pulmonary operation: the role of cardiopulmonary bypass. Ann Thorac Surg 1992;54(2):289–95.
37. Saxena P, Tam RK. Combined off-pump coronary artery bypass surgery and pulmonary resection. Ann Thorac Surg 2004;78:498–501.
38. Lu H, Wu Y, Hsieh M. Minimally invasive surgery for coronary artery disease with associated lung cancer. Chang Gung Med J 2002;25:110–4.
39. Rao V, Todd TR, Weisel RD, et al. Results of combined pulmonary resection and cardiac operation. Ann Thorac Surg 1996;62:342–7.
40. Mariani MA, Van Boven WJ, Duurkens VA, et al. Combined off-pump coronary surgery and right lung resections through midline sternotomy. Ann Thorac Surg 2001;71:1343–4.
41. Terzi A, Furlan G, Magnanelli G, et al. Lung resections concomitant to coronary artery bypass grafting. Eur J Cardiothorac Surg 1994;8:580–4.
42. Canver CC, Bhayana JN, Lajos TZ, et al. Pulmonary resection combined with cardiac operations. Ann Thorac Surg 1990;50:797–9.

43. Dyszkiewicz W, Jemielity M, Piwkowski C, et al. The early and late results of combined off-pump coronary artery bypass grafting and pulmonary resection in patients with concomitant lung cancer and unstable coronary heart disease. Eur J Cardiothorac Surg 2008;34:531–5.
44. Hosoba S, Hanaoka J, Suzuki T, et al. Early to midterm results of cardiac surgery with concomitant pulmonary resection. Ann Thorac Cardiovasc Surg 2012;18:8–11.
45. Yokoama T, Derrick M, Lee A. Cardiac operation with associated pulmonary resection. J Thorac Cardiovasc Surg 1993;105:912–5.
46. Kelpis T, Economopoulos V, Nikoloudakis N, et al. Minimally invasive transapical aortic valve implantation and simultaneous major pulmonary resection. J Card Surg 2013;28(6):660–2.
47. Thourani V, Borger M, Holmes D, et al. Transatlantic editorial on transcatheter aortic valve replacement. Ann Thorac Surg 2017;104:1–15.

Management of Malignant Lung Entrapment, the Oncothorax

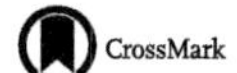

Roman Petrov, MD, Charles Bakhos, MD, Abbas E. Abbas, MD*

KEYWORDS

- Lung entrapment • Pleurectomy • Photodynamic therapy • Pleural catheter
- Hyperthermic chemoperfusion

KEY POINTS

- It is estimated that up to 30% of patients with advanced malignancy will have pleural metastasis, with lung cancer followed by breast and ovarian cancer the most common.
- The additional effect of lung entrapment causes the equivalent of a fibrothorax, indeed it is an "oncothorax."
- The standard approach for managing these patients is to place an indwelling catheter with the hope of preventing further compression of the lung by the fluid. However, this will not allow full reexpansion of the lung in most situations.

INTRODUCTION

Metastatic pleural disease is a tragic but relatively common occurrence in patients with most types of cancer. It is estimated that up to 30% of patients with advanced malignancy will have pleural metastasis, with lung cancer followed by breast and ovarian cancer the most common.[1] The presence of malignant pleural metastasis is almost always classified as distant metastasis or stage IV, even from ipsilateral lung cancer with the sole exception of mesothelioma, a primary malignancy of the pleura. A malignant pleural effusion (MPE) inevitably confers poor prognosis. In a meta-analysis of 417 patients with MPE, the median survival was 4 months, shortest for patients with lung cancer.[1] However, due to the often-incapacitating symptoms, including dyspnea, pain, and cough, the goal of therapy for this devastating disease should always focus on palliation of symptoms.

Usually, when MPE first occurs, it is a free-flowing collection that is not loculated. This can often be easily managed with simple thoracentesis or pleurodesis. However, much like its benign counterpart, with time, the lung may form adhesions to the lung, causing entrapment and loculation of the fluid. The additional effect of lung entrapment causes the equivalent of a fibrothorax, indeed it is an "oncothorax." This causes a restrictive lung disorder in addition to that caused by the malignant hydrothorax. Unfortunately, these adhesions that entrap the lung are often malignant and not typically amenable to surgical decortication. The standard approach for managing these patients is to place an indwelling catheter with the hope of preventing further compression of the lung by the fluid. However, this will not allow full reexpansion of the lung in most situations.

This article focuses on the unique situation of malignant lung entrapment from pleural metastasis. We use the term "oncothorax" to describe

Disclosure Statement: There are no disclosures or conflicts of interest.
Division of Thoracic Surgery, Department of Thoracic Medicine and Surgery, Temple University Hospital, Fox Chase Cancer Center, Lewis Katz School of Medicine, 3401 North Broad Street, Philadelphia, PA 19140, USA
* Corresponding author.
E-mail address: Abbas.Abbas@tuhs.temple.edu

Thorac Surg Clin 28 (2018) 81–90
https://doi.org/10.1016/j.thorsurg.2017.08.009

thoracic.theclinics.com

this phenomenon. To our knowledge, this name has not been previously used but does inherently describe the process and differentiates it from the more common MPE without entrapment of the lung. We present the therapeutic modalities available to manage this difficult syndrome.

PATHOPHYSIOLOGY

The pleural cavity contains a small amount of lubricating fluid (0.3 mL/kg body mass) between the visceral and parietal pleura under normal conditions.[2] This fluid is in continuous movement between the pleural membranes, and it is thought that the lymphatic system plays an important role in its homeostasis and balance.[3] The clearance of fluid within the pleural space is not fully understood, even though it is felt that fluid accumulation originates from the visceral pleura and is drained by the parietal pleura.[4] Transmission electron microscopy of human parietal pleura has also revealed the presence of lymphatic pleural stomata on the diaphragmatic surface of parietal pleura that serves to drain the pleural space of fluid and particles.[5,6] Malignancies can cause dysfunction of the pleural fluid flow dynamics and drainage by different means. First, obstruction of lymphatics or obstruction by enlarged mediastinal lymph nodes can increase the hydrostatic pressure of the interstitial tissue, leading to an increased fluid volume. Second, fluid absorption can be impaired by tumor involvement of the visceral and parietal pleura, inducing an inflammatory response and resulting in increased capillary permeability.[7] Third, cancers can also produce proliferative stimulants, such as cytokines, neurotransmitters, and growth factors that can promote pleural effusions.[8] Lung entrapment, or fibrothorax, occurs in long-standing benign pleural effusion from buildup of a fibrous layer of connective tissue over the collapsed lung, preventing its full reexpansion. This frequently results from inadequately treated parapneumonic effusions or empyema. This scenario is more challenging in mesothelioma or metastatic pleural disease, as the malignant pleural deposits tend to form effusions at a high volume. In addition, the adhesions that form are usually due to direct malignant invasion of the chest wall and lung. This combination of massive malignant effusion and malignant pleural rind will distort the respiratory mechanics by preventing normal chest wall excursion and enhancing the ventilation perfusion mismatch. A persistent pleural space due to lung atelectasis will invariably lead to further production of pleural fluid, thus perpetuating this vicious cycle.

DIAGNOSIS

Initial diagnosis of pleural effusion is usually based on chest radiography. A unilateral process should raise a high suspicion of malignancy or an infectious etiology. Computed tomography of the chest offers better resolution and anatomic definition of the process, showing a thick rind and fluid loculation, both of which are characteristic for entrapped lung (**Fig. 1**). Drainage of the fluid will confirm the latter, with lack of lung expansion and persistence of a pleural space. A thoracentesis is the least-invasive initial step to accomplish initial drainage, and the fluid is sent for analysis (cultures, cell count, cytology, and biochemical tests). A MPE or an infectious process will typically reveal an exudative pattern according to the criteria of Light and colleagues.[9] The sensitivity of thoracentesis and cytology to establish a diagnosis of malignancy ranges between 40% and 87%.[10,11] Repeat

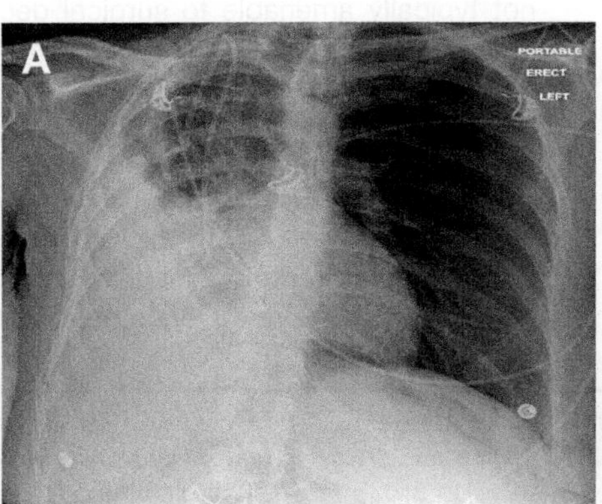

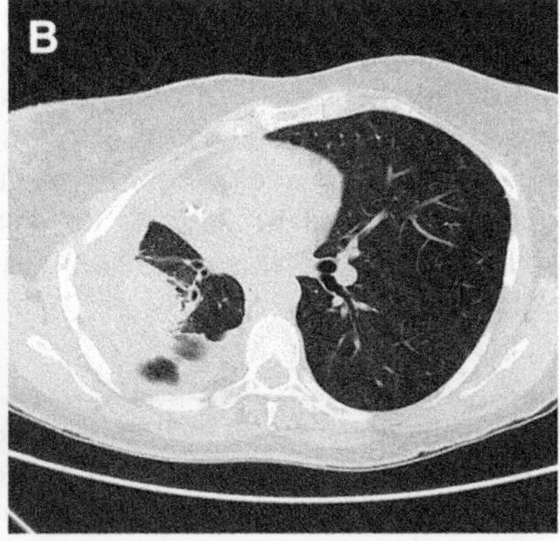

Fig. 1 (*A*) Chest radiograph and (*B*) computed tomography showing a chronic MPE and lung entrapment in a patient with history of metastatic ovarian cancer. Pleural thickening can be seen along with rounded atelectasis affecting all lobes and resulting in a contracted right hemithorax.

drainage and analysis may be required then, or alternatively, thoracoscopic exploration and pleural biopsies.

MANAGEMENT OF RECURRENT MALIGNANT PLEURAL EFFUSION

Most cases of MPE will recur within a month of drainage,[12] but a repeat thoracentesis can be considered in cases of slow reaccumulation and/or short life expectancy. Even though chemotherapy can help control a MPE in certain cancers (breast, small cell carcinoma of the lung, germ cell tumors, and lymphoma[13,14]), definitive management is usually required. This should take into account the functional status of the patients and their preferences, as well as the life expectancy, nutritional status, and tumor burden. As such, goals of therapy mostly focus on palliation of symptoms and providing comfort with minimization of hospitalization.

Pleurodesis

The goal of pleurodesis is to obliterate the pleural space by creating a seal between the visceral and parietal pleura, preventing reaccumulation of the effusion. Mechanical pleurodesis and induction of pleural abrasions are not typically recommended in malignant processes, mainly because of bleeding risk and high morbidity in terminally ill patients. Chemical pleurodesis can be performed using a variety of drugs, such as Adriamycin, tetracycline, doxycycline, bleomycin, talc, and even iodine.[15] Talc pleurodesis is a procedure that enjoys wide clinical applications. Initially introduced in the 1930s by Canadian thoracic surgeon Norman Bethune,[16] it induces a severe inflammatory and fibrotic response to multiple foreign bodies/talc particles.

Technique

Talc for pleurodesis can be used in the form of talc slurry via chest tube or as aerosolized insufflations (poudrage) during video-assisted thoracic surgery (VATS) (**Fig. 2**). The latter can be performed via a uniportal approach. On entrance of the pleural cavity, aerosolized talc spray can be used to disperse talc particles over the pleural lining. When talc is supplied in glass containers, it can be insufflated by connecting it to suction tubing and oxygen flow at 6 L per minute. That provides very even dispersion of the talc over pleural surfaces. The chest ports should be covered with wet towels to prevent contamination of the air.

Talc slurry is achieved by instilling suspension of 4 g of talc in 50 mL of normal saline through an already existing chest tube. A local anesthetic can be added in the mixture to help reduce the ensuing pain from pleurodesis. The procedure is performed at the bedside and the patient is encouraged to roll in bed for approximately 2 hours to assist in equal distribution of the talc over pleural surfaces. Not infrequently, the patient requires conscious sedation and/or close observation in a telemetry unit during and after the procedure.

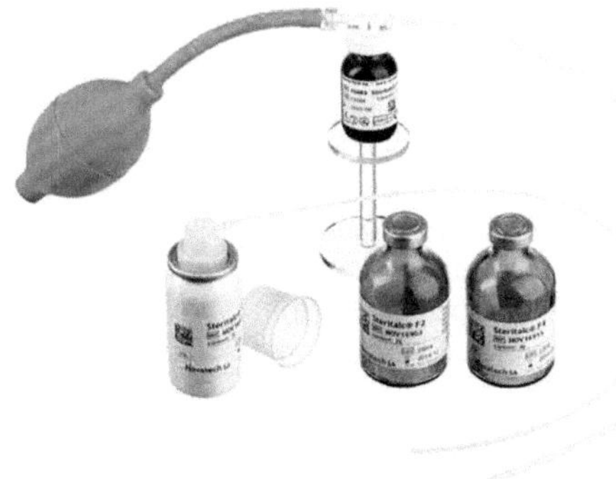

Fig. 2. Sterile talc in aerosolized spray and powder form. (© Novatech S.A, France.)

Results

In a randomized trial of 482 patients, Dresler and colleagues[17] demonstrated similar efficacy of talc slurry (71%) and thoracoscopic talc insufflation (TTI) (77%). However, subgroup analysis showed better results in patients with primary lung or breast cancer who underwent TTI (82% vs 67%), as defined by absence of effusion recurrence on imaging 30 days after the procedure. Additionally, quality of life appeared to be better in the TTI group. Similarly, the success rate has been reported as high as 93% in a series of 614 consecutive patients with pleural effusions who underwent thoracoscopic talc poudrage, although 11% of the patient population was excluded due to trapped lung or early death.[18] The most common adverse events following talc pleurodesis include fever and pain. More serious morbidity includes respiratory failure, reexpansion pulmonary edema, hypoxia, empyema, atrial fibrillation, and even death.[17,19] Furthermore, concerns were raised of the safety of talc regarding development of systemic inflammatory response syndrome (SIRS), acute respiratory distress syndrome (ARDS), and potential malignancy related to contamination with asbestos and particle size.[20] In fact, experimental animal models suggest systemic distribution of the talc after intrapleural administration.[21] In an analysis of clinical application of graded talc (with particles <10 nm removed) and mixed talc, Maskell and colleagues[22] demonstrated more SIRS and oxygen gradient in patients who received mixed. Additionally, Janssen and coauthors[23] conducted a large multicenter international study with inclusion of 550 patients with MPE. The investigators used 4 g of large-particle calibrated talc and reported no incidence of ARDS and a low rate of postoperative complications.[23]

The other chemical agents that have been used in pleurodesis include hypertonic saline, silver nitrate, nitrogen mustard, and sodium hydroxide.[24–26] However, in a meta-analysis of available literature, talc poudrage was found to be more effective in managing MPE than most other frequently used methods, including tetracycline and bleomycin.[27]

It is necessary that apposition of visceral and parietal plurae will occur for pleurodesis to be successful. This is rarely the case with oncothorax or malignant lung entrapment. It is therefore attempted only in the rare cases in which the surgeon was able to reexpand the lung after minor dissection.

INDWELLING PLEURAL CATHETER

Indwelling tunneled pleural catheters are a therapeutic alternative to recurrent MPE, and allow intermittent drainage on an outpatient basis. In cases of lung entrapment, they provide symptom palliation by preventing reaccumulation of the effusion, and they can help achieve pleural symphysis in cases of lung reexpansion. Two systems currently exist in the United States: the PleurX catheter (CareFusion, San Diego, CA), which uses a vacuum bottle, and the Aspira pleural catheter drainage system (Bard Access Systems, Salt Lake City, UT), which uses a low-vacuum siphon pump (**Fig. 3**).

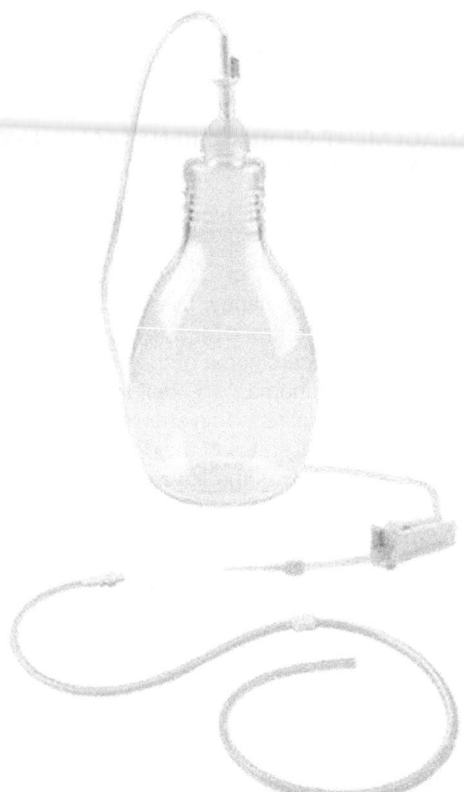

Fig. 3. Pleurx system, by carefusion. (*Courtesy* and © Becton, Dickinson and Company.)

Technique

Tunneled pleural catheters are placed percutaneously using a Seldinger technique and under ultrasound guidance, to best identify the pleural fluid pocket/area. Even though they can be performed at the bedside, we recommend an operative and strict sterile setting with monitored anesthesia care (MAC), with the patient in a mild decubitus position. In cases in which a sufficiently large fluid pocket cannot be identified, or early resistance is met when threading the wire or the peel-away sheath, concerns regarding the intrapleural location of the catheter are raised. In these cases, we advocate placing the catheter using VATS under either MAC or general anesthesia. After placement, drainage of the fluid should be stopped when the patient has a significant cough or air is encountered in the catheter itself. An airtight and sterile dressing is applied at the end. In cases of clogging, a solution of 10 to 20 mg tissue plasminogen activator can be instilled into the catheter to recanalize the lumen.

Results

In a randomized trial comparing indwelling pleural catheter to doxycycline pleurodesis, Putnam and colleagues[28] revealed excellent palliation of symptoms, a shorter median length of hospital stay (1.0 vs 6.5 days) and a lower rate of recurrence in the pleural catheter group. Another randomized trial of daily versus every other day drainage of indwelling pleural catheters in 149 patients demonstrated a higher rate of spontaneous pleurodesis (47% vs 24%) at an earlier date (54 vs 90 days), with no difference in the rate of adverse events.[29] Very high success rate as defined by improved dyspnea and/or quality of life has been reported by many retrospective series.[30–32] Similarly, a randomized prospective trial by Demmy and colleagues[33] compared bedside talc slurry with indwelling pleural catheter placement. The primary endpoint was combined success defined as consistent drainage/pleurodesis, lung expansion, and 30-day survival. The investigators found that combined success was higher with indwelling catheter than with bedside talc slurry (62% vs 46%, $P = .064$), and that patients who underwent catheter placement had a better survival with effusion control at 30 days compared with the pleurodesis group ($P = .024$). However, the trial had to be terminated early because of insufficient accrual (total n = 58 patients).[33]

A recent meta-analysis of 68 randomized trials showed that although pleurodesis is best at cessation of fluid production, indwelling pleural catheters may be better for patient-centered outcomes, particularly control of dyspnea.[27]

Adverse events include the risk of catheter track seeding with potential for local infection, empyema and metastases, or catheter dysfunction or blockage requiring thrombolysis and even possible fracture and retained material during bedside removal.[34,35]

Cost analysis comparing pleural catheters with pleurodesis is relatively difficult, as expenses should take into account not only the lower cost of initial catheter placement, but also later expenses related to visiting nurses and chronic drainage.[36] A recent analysis from the United Kingdom appears to favor indwelling pleural catheter over talc pleurodesis in patients with limited survival (<14 weeks).[37]

Indwelling Catheter and Pleurodesis

Thoracoscopy and tunneled pleural catheters are not mutually exclusive procedures, as both can be performed to achieve pleurodesis and potentially shorten the duration of hospitalization. Pleurodesis can be performed through the catheter with talc slurry, as reported by Ahmed and colleagues.[38] After instillation of 4 g of talc in 50 mL of normal saline, patients underwent daily drainage of the effusion. Based on ultrasound imaging, pleurodesis was achieved in 92% of patients 3 days after the procedure. At that point, drainage was held and catheter removed after 2 weeks. Similar success was reported in another series, in which a pleural catheter was placed during medical pleuroscopy and talc poudrage in 30 patients.[39]

PLEUROPERITONEAL SHUNT

Pleuroperitoneal shunts are rarely performed in the management of MPE, because indwelling tunneled catheters became available. They can still be used in cases of lung entrapment with inadequate lung expansion. In a large series, Genc and colleagues[40] placed pleuroperitoneal shunts thoracoscopically in 160 patients and reported a 95% successful palliation rate with 1.87% mortality and 14.8% complication rate. That included shunt occlusion requiring revision or replacement, skin erosion, and structural failure. Interestingly, tumor implants were reported at the site of insertion but not in the peritoneum.[40] Similar results were reported by other series, including tract seeding in cases of mesothelioma.[41,42]

MANAGEMENT OF MALIGNANT LUNG ENTRAPMENT (ONCOTHORAX)

Compared with benign empyema, management of malignant lung entrapment is particularly challenging. Patients are usually more debilitated, and both the parietal and visceral pleura can be involved with tumor infiltration, not only preventing lung expansion but also impairing chest wall excursion. Besides indwelling pleural catheters and pleuroperitoneal shunts, a few other therapeutic options are available in this scenario.

PLEURECTOMY AND DECORTICATION

Whereas entrapped lung in benign diseases develops as a result of fibrotic rind over the visceral pleura, it is usually due to infiltration and thickening of the visceral pleura in malignant processes.[43] Thus, the plane of dissection is deeper and involves removal of the visceral pleura. This procedure is more widely accepted in the treatment of malignant mesothelioma as an alternative to extrapleural pneumonectomy.[44] It is usually of less value in the setting of metastatic pleural disease due to limited expected survival and poor patient condition from advanced malignancy and systemic effects of antitumor therapy.

Technique

A pleurectomy decortication is performed with the patient in lateral decubitus position, under general anesthesia and lung isolation. Using the VATS approach, the initial port can be placed anterior and inferior to the scapular tip, or in the fourth to fifth intercostal space in the midaxillary line, potentially away from the disease process. Digital exploration can help free adhesions and avoid parenchymal tears on first entry, and the other 2 ports are placed under direct camera vision. Alternatively, a single-port approach can be used with the 30° camera and curved instruments fitting through a 2.5-cm anterior incision in the sixth or seventh intercostal space. A wound protector is used to retract the subcutaneous and muscle tissue. Pleural fluid is initially drained and the decortication is carried in a similar fashion to an empyema. The visceral pleura is incised with endoscopic shears and carefully peeled off from the underlying trapped lung. This can be achieved using blunt dissection with a peanut dissector or the Yankauer suction tip. A thick cortex can be held with a Kocher device, and gynecologic curettes can sometimes be helpful to follow and extend the plane of dissection. Intermittent continuous positive airway pressure can be applied to the operative lung to facilitate the dissection. The goal is to allow adequate lung expansion and apposition of the parenchyma against the chest wall. A partial or even a subtotal pleurectomy/decortication can be achieved with the VATS approach, but an extended pleurectomy decortication with removal of the diaphragm and pericardium usually necessitates a posterolateral thoracotomy, extending anteriorly and inferiorly. This is particularly true in cases of malignant mesothelioma, in which the goal of surgery is to achieve a complete macroscopic resection and improve survival in fit patients with reasonable life expectancy. The sixth rib is removed and the parietal pleura dissected in an extrapleural plane using finger blunt dissection (**Fig. 4**). After placement of the Finochietto chest retractor, dissection is carried to the apex with special care not to injure major vessels, and the mediastinal pleura mobilized with a peanut sponge. The diaphragm is then mobilized by freeing its insertion from the chest wall, and cautery used in the dissection plane from lateral to medial. Reconstruction of the diaphragm is performed with 2-mm-thick polytetrafluoroethylene mesh. Decortication of the visceral pleura is carried with a needle tip cautery, with care to clear the tumor burden down to the fissures. If the pleura is attached to the pericardium, the latter is excised and the ensuing defect closed with absorbable mesh. Adequate chest tube drainage is essential to ensure full expansion of the lung and avoid space problems.

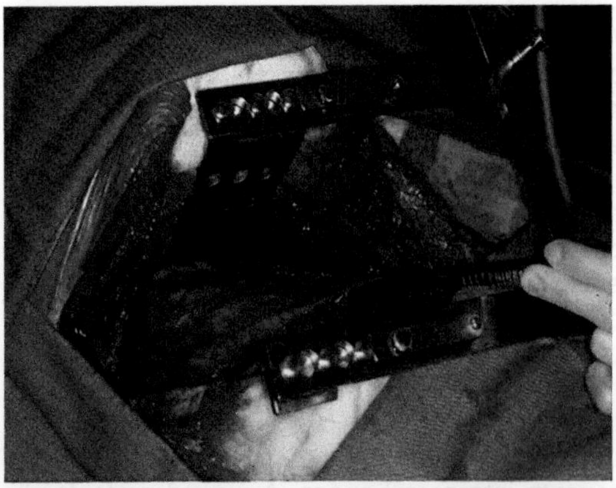

Fig. 4. The parietal pleura being mobilized away from the chest wall and the endothoracic fascia, in a patient with malignant pleural mesothelioma. (*From* Rusch VW. Pleurectomy and decortication: how I teach it. Ann Thorac Surg 2017;103(5):1378; with permission.)

Results

Benefits of visceral pleurectomy include lung reexpansion and improvement of hypoxia and ventilation perfusion mismatch. In fact, persistent lung expansion has been demonstrated by Sensakovic and colleagues,[45] where 83% of patients with mesothelioma achieved 44% increase in their lung volumes until at least 4 months after the intervention. Approximately a similar percentage of patients with mesothelioma achieved significant improvement in pulmonary function tests, especially when the diaphragm was preserved.[46] However, the impact of pleurectomy on survival was not demonstrated in the mesoVATS study, in which 175 patients with mesothelioma and pleural effusion were randomly assigned to VATS partial pleurectomy (VATS-PP) or talc pleurodesis. The overall survival at 1 year was in fact similar between the 2 groups (52% vs 57%, respectively), but surgical complications and pulmonary complications (including prolonged air leak) were significantly more prevalent in the VATS-PP group.[47]

DECORTICATION WITH INTRAOPERATIVE HYPERTHERMIC CHEMOPERFUSION

Most treatment modalities of MPE and metastatic disease are palliative in nature, and do not confer a survival benefit. Intraoperative chemoperfusion represent a paradigm shift in managing these patients, and the procedure can be done in conjunction with decortication and pleurectomy if indicated. The interest for intraoperative chemotherapy was sparked by Dedrick and colleagues[48] in 1978. The rationale for local administration of chemotherapy agents is potential dose escalation with limited systemic absorption and toxicity. In fact, intrapleural cisplatin administration has been shown to be associated with lower plasma concentrations compared with the pleural cavity, even more so if a pleurectomy is performed. This is presumed to be due to the absorptive properties of the pleura.[49,50] Furthermore, hyperthermia as high as 44°C can potentiate the cytotoxic effect of drugs, overcome chemoresistance, and promote apoptosis of cancer cells, without causing much harm.[51]

Technique

At the completion of pleurectomy via VATS or thoracotomy, preparation is made for chemoperfusion. The chest is inspected to determine the degree of residual disease. Incomplete resection with presence of tumor fragments larger than 2 cm is usually considered a contraindication for intrapleural chemoperfusion. Retractors are removed and an occlusive adhesive drape is placed over the incisions. Inflow and outflow catheters are introduced through the drape and infusion of the chest with the agent (usually cisplatin diluted in saline) at a temperature of 42.0 to 45°C for 60 to 90 minutes (**Fig. 5**). Sodium thiosulfate can be administered intravenously to limit the systemic absorption and provide renal protection whenever cisplatin is used. In addition, urine output is maintained at ≥100 mL/h during chemotherapy infusion using intravenous fluids, furosemide, and/or mannitol. Patient body temperature is monitored with an esophageal temperature probe; cooling blankets and/or ice packs are used if necessary to maintain body temperature lower than 40°C. An additional temperature probe is placed into the thorax to confirm a continuous temperature of the perfusion solution. At the completion of perfusion, all fluid is suctioned out of the thorax, which is irrigated with normal saline.

Results

The effect of intraoperative hyperthermic chemoperfusion on survival has been thoroughly reported. Sugarbaker and colleagues[52] showed a longer interval to recurrence and improved survival in 103 low-risk patients with malignant pleural mesothelioma who underwent extrapleural pneumonectomy. This modality also can be applied in lung cancer with pleural dissemination, as reported by Yi and colleagues.[53] The investigators used a 90-minute perfusion of 150 mg/m^2 of cisplatin with mannitol and thiosulphate protection at 43 to 45°C. There was statistically significant improvement of overall survival at 6 months, 1 year, and 3 years (95.7%, 91.3%, and 38.6% vs 80.0%, 80.0%, and 37.5%) and trend toward improved progression-free survival (87.0%, 47.8%, and 24.3%, vs 44.4%, 33.3%, and 0.0%). No mortality was noted in that series. Other applications of hyperthermic pleural lavage include stage IV thymoma with pleural dissemination.[54] Future technologies involve immobilizing chemotherapy agents on carrier molecules to increase the intrapleural concentration and duration of exposure, therefore reducing systemic reabsorption.[55,56]

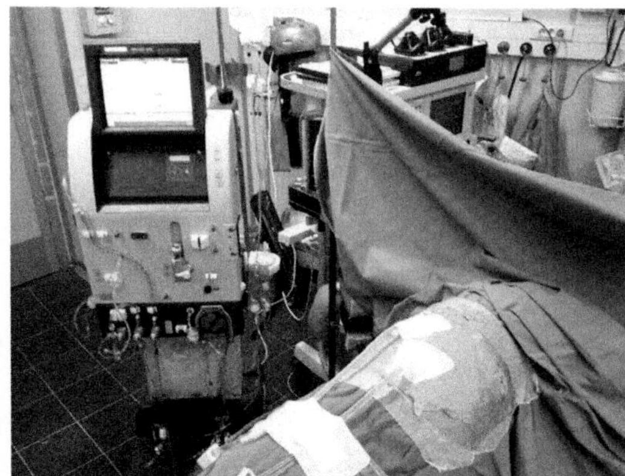

Fig. 5. The patient is connected to the extracorporeal circulation circuit to apply hyperthermic pleural chemoperfusion, with an inflow and outflow chest drain. (*From* Asteriou C, Kleontas A, Barbetakis N. Recent advances in surgical techniques for multimodality treatment of malignant pleural mesothelioma. In: Firstenberg MS, editor. Principles and practice of cardiothoracic surgery. Rijekak (Croatia): Intech; 2013. p. 167–93; with permission.)

INTRAPLEURAL PHOTODYNAMIC THERAPY

Having a long-standing history in the treatment of endoluminal esophageal and lung cancer, photodynamic therapy (PDT) has recently been proposed for the management of pleural disease in patients with malignant mesothelioma. A light-based treatment, PDT consists of 3 components: a nontoxic porphyrin-based photosensitizing agent, oxygen, and visible light. It is believed that PDT can directly kill cancer cells, destroy the tumor neovasculature, and induce a tumor-directed immune response.[57] Because the visible light penetrates several millimeters into tissue, PDT will treat for a short depth below the surface. Encouraging results were reported by Friedberg and colleagues[58] in 38 patients with stage III/IV mesothelioma who underwent lung-sparing pleurectomy and intraoperative PDT. The overall median survival was 31.7 months (41.2 months for epithelial type), which is superior to results reported in many surgical series, especially in patients with such advanced disease. Similarly, Chen and colleagues[59] used PDT and radical surgical resection in 18 patients with malignant pleural disease (lungs n = 10 and thymoma n = 8). There was no procedure-related mortality, and the 3-year and 5-year survival were as high as 68.9% and 57.4%. In a study by Chen and colleagues[59] of 51 patients who underwent intrapleural PDT for metastatic pleural disease from metastatic lung and thymic cancer, the median survival of patients with lung cancer who underwent PDT was better than those who had chemotherapy or targeted therapy (39.0 vs 17.6 months).

Although the experience with PDT in pleural disease is limited, it appears that the technology may help control residual microscopic disease after radical resection. Further work is needed to better clarify its role in clinical practice.

THE INFECTED ONCOTHORAX

Although rare, a loculated malignant effusion may become superinfected, especially if drainage interventions have been attempted. This may cause a pleural abscess and lead to severe sepsis. This situation in benign disease is normally managed by drainage and decortication; however, in malignant entrapment, the lung is unlikely to reexpand after drainage or decortication, leaving a chronic space that will be a nidus for recurrence.

Our approach to this difficult situation is to attempt closed catheter drainage and instillation of antibiotics. If this fails to resolve the ongoing infection (and the patient can tolerate surgery), it may be warranted to perform a pleurectomy for decortication with muscle flap coverage of any residual space (modified Clagett procedure).[60] In cases of MPE, any attempt at creating a permanent drainage window (Eloesser flap) may be complicated by massive drainage and skin seeding.

SUMMARY AND RECOMMENDATIONS

Development of metastatic pleural disease with trapped lung (oncothorax) is usually extremely debilitating in patients with a limited prognosis. Traditional options for free-flowing MPE, such as thoracentesis or pleurodesis, are not reasonable options because pleural apposition is necessary for development of pleural symphysis. Placement of an indwelling catheter lately has been the primary modality used in these situations. Although it does not address fluid production, it may partially palliate dyspnea and allow transition of the patient to independent home care.

There are currently new approaches available, such as pleurectomy and intraoperative hyperthermic chemoperfusion, which have been occasionally offered with curative intent. However, these procedures are complex, require significant expertise, and can be applied only to a very select group of patients with excellent performance status, controlled primary disease, established disease-free interval, and localized unilateral metastases. They should be performed preferably within the confines of clinical trials and in centers with significant expertise.

REFERENCES

1. Heffner JE, Nietert PJ, Barbieri C. Pleural fluid pH as a predictor of pleurodesis failure: analysis of primary data. Chest 2000;117(1):87–95.
2. Miserocchi G. Physiology and pathophysiology of pleural fluid turnover. Eur Respir J 1997;10(1): 219–25.
3. Miserocchi G, Venturoli D, Negrini D, et al. Intrapleural fluid movements described by a porous flow model. J Appl Physiol (1985) 1992;73(6):2511–6.
4. English JC, Leslie KO. Pathology of the pleura. Clin Chest Med 2000;27(2):157–80.
5. Li J, Jiang B. A scanning electron microscopic study on three-dimensional organization of human diaphragmatic lymphatics. Funct Dev Morphol 1993; 3(2):129–32.
6. Peng MJ, Wang NS, Vargas FS, et al. Subclinical surface alterations of human pleura. A scanning electron microscopic study. Chest 1994;106(2): 351–3.
7. DeCamp MM Jr, Mentzer SJ, Swanson SJ, et al. Malignant effusive disease of the pleura and pericardium. Chest 1997;112(4 Suppl):291S–5S.
8. Kassis J, Klominek J, Kohn EC. Tumor microenvironment: what can effusions teach us? Diagn Cytopathol 2005;33(5):316–9.
9. Light RW, Macgregor MI, Luchsinger PC, et al. Pleural effusions: The diagnostic separation of transudates and exudates. Ann Intern Med 1972;77(4): 507–13.
10. Jay SJ. Diagnostic procedures for pleural disease. Clin Chest Med 1985;6(1):33–48.
11. Toms AP, Tasker AD, Flower CD. Intervention in the pleura. Eur J Radiol 2000;34(2):119–32.
12. Antunes G, Neville E, Duffy J, et al, Pleural Diseases Group, Standards of Care Committee, British Thoracic Society. BTS guidelines for the management of malignant pleural effusions. Thorax 2003; 58(Suppl 2):ii29–38.
13. Weick JK, Kiely JM, Harrison EG Jr, et al. Pleural effusion in lymphoma. Cancer 1973;31(4):848–53.
14. Livingston RB, McCracken JD, Trauth CJ, et al. Isolated pleural effusion in small cell lung carcinoma: favorable prognosis. A review of the Southwest Oncology Group experience. Chest 1982;81(2): 208–11.
15. Shaw P, Agarwal R. Pleurodesis for malignant pleural effusions. Cochrane Database Syst Rev 2004;(1):CD002916.
16. Bethune N. Pleural poudrage: new technique for the deliberate production of pleural adhesion as preliminary to lobectomy. J Thorac Surg 1935;4:251–61.
17. Dresler CM, Olak J, Herndon JE 2nd, et al. Phase III intergroup study of talc poudrage vs talc slurry sclerosis for malignant pleural effusion. Chest 2005; 127(3):909–15.
18. de Campos JR, Vargas FS, de Campos Werebe E, et al. Thoracoscopy talc poudrage: a 15-year experience. Chest 2001;119(3):801–6.
19. Kennedy L, Rusch VW, Strange C, et al. Pleurodesis using talc slurry. Chest 1994;106(2):342–6.
20. Light RW. Talc should not be used for pleurodesis. Am J Respir Crit Care Med 2000;162(6): 2024–6.

21. Stamatelopoulos A, Koullias G, Arnaouti M, et al. Malignant pleural effusion and talc pleurodesis. experimental model regarding early kinetics of talc particle dissemination in the chest after experimental talc pleurodesis. J BUON 2009;14(3):419–23.
22. Maskell NA, Lee YC, Gleeson FV, et al. Randomized trials describing lung inflammation after pleurodesis with talc of varying particle size. Am J Respir Crit Care Med 2004;170(4):377–82.
23. Janssen JP, Collier G, Astoul P, et al. Safety of pleurodesis with talc poudrage in malignant pleural effusion: a prospective cohort study. Lancet 2007; 369(9572):1535–9.
24. Marchi E, Vargas FS, Teixeira LR, et al. Intrapleural low-dose silver nitrate elicits more pleural inflammation and less systemic inflammation than low-dose talc. Chest 2005;128(3):1798–804.
25. Paschoalini Mda S, Vargas FS, Marchi E, et al. Prospective randomized trial of silver nitrate vs talc slurry in pleurodesis for symptomatic malignant pleural effusions. Chest 2005;128(2):684–9.
26. Vargas FS, Carmo AO, Teixeira LR. A new look at old agents for pleurodesis: nitrogen mustard, sodium hydroxide, and silver nitrate. Curr Opin Pulm Med 2000;6(4):281–6.
27. Clive AO, Jones HE, Bhatnagar R, et al. Interventions for the management of malignant pleural effusions: a network meta-analysis. Cochrane Database Syst Rev 2016;(5):CD010529.
28. Putnam JB Jr, Light RW, Rodriguez RM, et al. A randomized comparison of indwelling pleural catheter and doxycycline pleurodesis in the management of malignant pleural effusions. Cancer 1999;86(10):1992–9.
29. Wahidi MM, Reddy C, Yarmus L, et al. Randomized trial of pleural fluid drainage frequency in patients with malignant pleural effusions. the ASAP trial. Am J Respir Crit Care Med 2017;195(8):1050–7.
30. Tremblay A, Michaud G. Single-center experience with 250 tunnelled pleural catheter insertions for malignant pleural effusion. Chest 2006;129(2):362–8.
31. Fysh ET, Waterer GW, Kendall PA, et al. Indwelling pleural catheters reduce inpatient days over pleurodesis for malignant pleural effusion. Chest 2012; 142(2):394–400.
32. Davies HE, Mishra EK, Kahan BC, et al. Effect of an indwelling pleural catheter vs chest tube and talc pleurodesis for relieving dyspnea in patients with malignant pleural effusion: The TIME2 randomized controlled trial. JAMA 2012;307(22):2383–9.
33. Demmy TL, Gu L, Burkhalter JE, et al. Optimal management of malignant pleural effusions (results of CALGB 30102). J Natl Compr Canc Netw 2012; 10(8):975–82.
34. Janes SM, Rahman NM, Davies RJ, et al. Catheter-tract metastases associated with chronic indwelling pleural catheters. Chest 2007;131(4):1232–4.
35. Fysh ET, Tremblay A, Feller-Kopman D, et al. Clinical outcomes of indwelling pleural catheter-related pleural infections: an international multicenter study. Chest 2013;144(5):1597–602.
36. MacEachern P, Tremblay A. Pleural controversy: pleurodesis versus indwelling pleural catheters for malignant effusions. Respirology 2011;16(5): 747–54.
37. Penz ED, Mishra EK, Davies HE, et al. Comparing cost of indwelling pleural catheter vs talc pleurodesis for malignant pleural effusion. Chest 2014; 146(4):991–1000.
38. Ahmed L, Ip H, Rao D, et al. Talc pleurodesis through indwelling pleural catheters for malignant pleural effusions: retrospective case series of a novel clinical pathway. Chest 2014;146(6):e190–4.
39. Reddy C, Ernst A, Lamb C, et al. Rapid pleurodesis for malignant pleural effusions: a pilot study. Chest 2011;139(6):1419–23.
40. Genc O, Petrou M, Ladas G, et al. The long-term morbidity of pleuroperitoneal shunts in the management of recurrent malignant effusions. Eur J Cardiothorac Surg 2000;18(2):143–6.
41. Tsang V, Fernando HC, Goldstraw P. Pleuroperitoneal shunt for recurrent malignant pleural effusions. Thorax 1990;45(5):369–72.
42. Baeyens I, Berrisford RG. Pleuroperitoneal shunts and tumor seeding. J Thorac Cardiovasc Surg 2001;121(4):813.
43. Rathinam S, Waller DA. Pleurectomy decortication in the treatment of the "trapped lung" in benign and malignant pleural effusions. Thorac Surg Clin 2013; 23(1):51–61, vi.
44. Rusch VW. Pleurectomy and decortication: how I teach it. Ann Thorac Surg 2017;103(5):1374–7.
45. Sensakovic WF, Armato SG 3rd, Starkey A, et al. Quantitative measurement of lung reexpansion in malignant pleural mesothelioma patients undergoing pleurectomy/decortication. Acad Radiol 2011; 18(3):294–8.
46. Bolukbas S, Eberlein M, Schirren J. Prospective study on functional results after lung-sparing radical pleurectomy in the management of malignant pleural mesothelioma. J Thorac Oncol 2012;7(5): 900–5.
47. Rintoul RC, Ritchie AJ, Edwards JG, et al. Efficacy and cost of video-assisted thoracoscopic partial pleurectomy versus talc pleurodesis in patients with malignant pleural mesothelioma (MesoVATS): an open-label, randomised, controlled trial. Lancet 2014;384(9948):1118–27.
48. Dedrick RL, Myers CE, Bungay PM, et al. Pharmacokinetic rationale for peritoneal drug administration in the treatment of ovarian cancer. Cancer Treat Rep 1978;62(1):1–11.
49. Rusch VW, Niedzwiecki D, Tao Y, et al. Intrapleural cisplatin and mitomycin for malignant mesothelioma

following pleurectomy: pharmacokinetic studies. J Clin Oncol 1992;10(6):1001–6.
50. Yasumoto K, Shimokawa T, Nagashima A, et al. Pharmacokinetics of cisplatin instilled into the pleural cavity following panpleuropneumonectomy in patients with malignant pleurisy due to lung cancer. J Surg Oncol 1993;54(2):67–70.
51. Zhang H, Zhan C, Ke J, et al. EGFR kinase domain mutation positive lung cancers are sensitive to intrapleural perfusion with hyperthermic chemotherapy (IPHC) complete treatment. Oncotarget 2016;7(3):3367–78.
52. Sugarbaker DJ, Gill RR, Yeap BY, et al. Hyperthermic intraoperative pleural cisplatin chemotherapy extends interval to recurrence and survival among low-risk patients with malignant pleural mesothelioma undergoing surgical macroscopic complete resection. J Thorac Cardiovasc Surg 2013;145(4):955–63.
53. Yi E, Kim D, Cho S, et al. Clinical outcomes of cytoreductive surgery combined with intrapleural perfusion of hyperthermic chemotherapy in advanced lung adenocarcinoma with pleural dissemination. J Thorac Dis 2016;8(7):1550–60.
54. Belcher E, Hardwick T, Lal R, et al. Induction chemotherapy, cytoreductive surgery and intraoperative hyperthermic pleural irrigation in patients with stage IVA thymoma. Interact Cardiovasc Thorac Surg 2011;12(5):744–7.
55. Opitz I, Erne BV, Demirbas S, et al. Optimized intrapleural cisplatin chemotherapy with a fibrin carrier after extrapleural pneumonectomy: a preclinical study. J Thorac Cardiovasc Surg 2011;141(1):65–71.
56. Lardinois D, Jung FJ, Opitz I, et al. Intrapleural topical application of cisplatin with the surgical carrier vivostat increases the local drug concentration in an immune-competent rat model with malignant pleuromesothelioma. J Thorac Cardiovasc Surg 2006;131(3):697–703.
57. Castano AP, Mroz P, Hamblin MR. Photodynamic therapy and anti-tumour immunity. Nat Rev Cancer 2006;6(7):535–45.
58. Friedberg JS, Culligan MJ, Mick R, et al. Radical pleurectomy and intraoperative photodynamic therapy for malignant pleural mesothelioma. Ann Thorac Surg 2012;93(5):1658–65 [discussion: 1665–7].
59. Chen KC, Hsieh YS, Tseng YF, et al. Pleural photodynamic therapy and surgery in lung cancer and thymoma patients with pleural spread. PLoS One 2015;10(7):e0133230.
60. Abbas A, Deschamps C. Postpneumonectomy empyema. Curr Opin Pulm Med 2002;8(4):327–33.

Empyema from Obstructing Lung Cancer

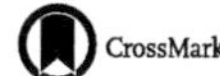

Julian Guitron, MD

KEYWORDS

- Obstructing cancer • Pleural effusion • Empyema • Malignant effusions • Para-malignant effusion

KEY POINTS

- It is of critical importance to fully investigate any pleural collection ipsilateral to an obstructing lung cancer.
- The order in which to approach patients is determined by presenting symptoms (pleural vs bronchial).
- A multidisciplinary approach is optimal when managing such complex patients.

INTRODUCTION

Pleural effusions that accompany obstructing lung cancers pose a particular challenge. In most situations, symptoms demand intervention; but in this situation, determining the nature of the effusion plays a critical role in the staging process. The fluid collection alone places patients in either stage IB if not malignant or stage IV if cancerous. It is, therefore, of paramount importance to place significant importance on determining the nature of the effusion and not rush to consider it a malignant-effusion and commit patients to a nonsurgical treatment modality. In this article, the author reviews the general principles of pleural effusions, including empyema, and their management with particular attention to those related to an obstructing mass.

PLEURAL CONDITIONS

The pleural space is a dynamic compartment of complex interactions between the parietal and visceral layers producing and reabsorbing pleural fluid at a rate of approximately 700 mL/d.[1] Any disturbance of that pleural balance will result in excess fluid accumulation, which over time can become infected. Alternatively, the fluid collection develops septations, resulting in a complex collection that ultimately traps the lung if left unattended. Approximately 50% of patients with metastatic malignancies develop a pleural effusion, including both malignant and para-malignant.[2]

Other pleural collections, such a chylothorax, are beyond the scope if this article but should always be considered when approaching patients with a malignancy and an unexplained pleural effusion.

Para-Malignant Effusion

With increasing diagnostic modalities and sensitivities over the past several years, it has become more frequent to diagnose para-malignant effusions. They are defined as benign fluid collections in the setting of a malignancy within the bronchial tree. These effusions pose a singular challenge when present in the ipsilateral side of the primary malignancy, as their appropriate diagnosis impacts the staging of the cancer dramatically. Patients may harbor either a small and localized cancer that obstructs a segmental bronchus with a simple mechanical process resulting in a pleural effusion (stage I) or a tumor with pleural dissemination resulting in a malignant effusion (stage IV). It is, therefore, of paramount importance to make every

Disclosure: The author has no conflicts of interest or financial disclosures pertaining to the article presented.
Section of Thoracic Surgery, ML0558, 234 Goodman Drive, Cincinnati, OH 45219, USA
E-mail address: Julian.guitron@uc.edu

Thorac Surg Clin 28 (2018) 91–96
https://doi.org/10.1016/j.thorsurg.2017.09.001

effort to establish the nature of the pleural effusion before committing patients to any treatment pathway.

Malignant Effusion

Any pleural effusion associated with a lung mass or any known cancer elsewhere should raise the concern of metastatic spread. This has prognostic implications, as the median survival of patients diagnosed with a malignant effusion is 4 months.[3] The typical malignant effusion is exudative, with only a minority being transudative. This initial finding of transudate fluid could indicate a paramalignant nature of the effusion encouraging further workup of the fluid to confirm its cause.[4] Initial imaging studies often demonstrates pleural implants that further raise suspicion of metastatic disease. Even in those circumstances, tissue confirmation is essential.

A thoracentesis is the ideal initial invasive approach to the effusion providing valuable information on the nature of the fluid itself as well as samples for microbiologic studies and cytologic analysis. This first step could establish the diagnosis of malignancy and avoid any further diagnostic interventions. Additionally, draining the pleural space provides symptomatic relief to patients with the potential added benefit of improving the performance status for further preoperative physiologic testing.

Trapped Lung

A prolonged presence of a pleural collection often results in trapped lung that does not re-expand despite the complete evacuation of the fluid. This condition results from a rind or peel that progressively forms over the visceral pleura that thickens over time. The resulting condition on completing a thoracentesis in this situation is an ex vacuo pneumothorax or hydropneumothorax if incompletely drained. Pleural manometry at the time of the thoracentesis can further differentiate the condition of the unexpandable lung into either trapped lung or lung entrapment.[5] Trapped lung refers to the unexpandable lung due to a thickened visceral pleura in the absence of an active pleural process. In other words, the parapneumonic effusion, empyema, or hemothorax resolved over time leaving behind the unexpanded lung that requires decortication to be re-expanded. Lung entrapment refers to an active pleural process that has resulted in the unexpanded lung. In this situation, the lung could re-expand if the active pleural process is treated promptly. Pleural manometry helps in the differentiation of these two conditions based on the pressure measurement at the time of the thoracentesis. In general, a sudden drop of the pleural pressure to less than 20 mm Hg indicates a trapped lung, whereas a gradual decrease of such negative pressure reflects entrapment, giving reasonable expectations that the lung could re-expand if the active pleural condition is treated successfully. The definitive criteria to distinguish both conditions by manometry are still being studied and are beyond the scope of this article. Nonetheless, gaining insight into the nature of a trapped lung versus lung entrapment helps determine which patients should be promptly referred for pleural decortication or, rather, be aggressively treated for the pleural process with the expectation that the lung will re-expand without surgical intervention.

MANAGEMENT OPTIONS

Any pleural process that results in fluid accumulation is likely to impact on patients' performance status and, therefore, requires intervention. Draining the pleural cavity accomplishes several goals, including relief of symptoms as well as establishing the nature of the effusion. Occasionally, it also establishes the diagnosis and results in the re-expansion of the lung. There are several pleural interventions available that, in general, are applied from least to most invasive.

Chest Tube Drainage

The initial thoracentesis often provides sufficient information that allows the clinician to decide if the placement of a pleural drain is warranted. With the needle in the pleural cavity, it is possible to pass a guidewire followed by a pigtail catheter. Over time it has become more common to start with a small-bore catheter even in the face of empyema, only upsizing to a bigger tube if needed.[6] The fluid is then sent for chemical, microbiological, and cytology studies.

Pleural Fibrinolytic Therapy

An untreated pleural effusion, particularly empyema, will frequently evolve into a loculated or compartmentalized collection. In this setting, a single drain is often ineffective in resolving the process. Traditionally, this was an indication for surgical drainage. However, the use of fibrinolytics in the pleural space has shown significant effectiveness in lysing loculations and thinning the fluid with good results. The results of a randomized trial comparing placebo versus both tissue plasminogen activator and deoxyribonuclease were published in 2011.[7] The combined therapy demonstrated increased effectiveness in draining complex collections and decreased the need of surgical intervention. The author and colleagues adopted that protocol at their institution with good results consistent with the trial outcomes. Their practice is to administer the fibrinolytic mixture every 12 hours, 3 times followed by computed tomography (CT) scan reassessment of the chest once the volume of output has decreased. Based on the imaging findings, they can determine if further intervention is needed, including additional doses of fibrinolytics or surgical exploration and drainage.

Pleurodesis

There are several techniques that result in the fusion of the pleural surfaces to prevent recurrent pneumothorax or fluid collections. Common to all of them is the absolute requirement that both visceral and parietal pleural surfaces meet, allowing the formation of adhesions and ultimately scar tissue that will withstand the pressures exerted by air of the fluid. Pleurodesis can be induced through an already placed chest tube if there is evidence that the lung expands when suction is applied on a chest radiograph. A talc slurry is typically prepared and should be administered promptly to avoid precipitation. In most instances, the chest tube is clamped for approximately an hour to allow the talc to induce the inflammatory response that is needed. This process typically elicits significant pain; therefore, a pain management strategy has to be in place. The author and colleagues often use epidural analgesia in this situation. Once the chest tube is unclamped, suction is applied for uninterrupted 48 to 72 hours. Recently, the Food and Drug Administration approved the application of a talc slurry through a tunneled pleural catheter. This practice benefits patients who have a tunneled catheter in place but do not achieve spontaneous pleurodesis, which has been described as high as 70% within 2 to 6 weeks after placing the catheter.[8,9] When the diagnosis has not been established, a medical pleuroscopy or a VATS exploration are ideal to provide directed biopsy specimens, which often can be assessed on frozen pathologic assessment. If malignancy is confirmed, a talc mixture can be applied under direct visualization achieving superior results compared with chest tube-directed application.[10] In cases whereby no malignancy is involved, a mechanical pleurodesis is preferred by ablating the parietal pleural surface during video-assisted thoracoscopic surgery (VATS) exploration.

Pleural Exploration

Every effort should be made to determine the nature of a fluid collection in the setting of an endobronchial malignancy. Often cytologic assessment of the fluid is not conclusive; therefore, pleural exploration should be considered. Patients with limited physiologic reserves may undergo a medical pleuroscopy. Individuals with suspected trapped lung should be considered for a VATS or open exploration for biopsy and decortication if malignancy is ruled out.

Medical Pleuroscopy

In patients with limited physiologic reserves, particularly those who would not tolerate single-lung ventilation or general anesthesia, medical pleuroscopy should be considered. Patients are positioned in lateral decubitus and sedation is induced, and the ultrasound is used to mark the ideal place for the 4- to 5-mm trocar. Ideally, the site of a fluid collection is chosen, although in the author's experience, the visualization of sliding pleural surfaces is sufficient evidence for a safe pleural entry even in the absence of an effusion. Local anesthetic is infiltrated, particularly at the subpleural level, followed by a subcentimeter incision. The 4-mm trocar is then placed, and some of the fluid is suctioned out and sent for various tests. Scopes with several angulations are then used to assess the pleura and identify targets for biopsy. Biopsy forceps are then coupled with the scopes, allowing sampling under direct visualization. This approach further facilitates the takedown of adhesions and thorough draining of the pleural space. A small-bore chest tube is then placed on suction and typically removed the following morning.

Video-Assisted Thoracoscopic Surgery and Open Explorations

The overall condition of patients determines the level of invasiveness that is most appropriate for the clinical situation. Single-lung ventilation and general anesthesia are two of the most important considerations. Often, the nature of the pleural process itself has rendered patients physiologically on single-lung ventilation; therefore, tolerance for a more invasive approach should be considered. Lung isolation allows for the placement of additional ports and the use of larger instruments that facilitate the takedown of adhesions and drainage of the pleural cavity. Furthermore, decortication is possible via the VATS approach. Nonetheless, if malignancy is confirmed on frozen section, the pleural intervention is minimized and focus is directed toward quality of life.

Exploration via thoracotomy, most often through a posterolateral approach, will provide the exposure and access necessary to resolve most benign cases. The endobronchial obstructing tumor must be kept in mind when deciding on proceeding with a thoracotomy, as often patients will benefit from endobronchial debridement of the tumors to open the airway followed by induction therapy depending on the clinical stage of the malignancy. Once completed, the thoracotomy approach is ideal not only to provide adequate exposure but also to procure a pedicled muscle flap to buttress the bronchial stump.

An empyema with trapped lung traditionally requires an open thoracostomy window. However, the morbidity of an Eloesser flap and Clagett process may be prohibitive to debilitated patients undergoing chemotherapy or presenting unresectable disease. Therefore, alternative treatment modalities should be considered. Options include fibrinolytic therapy alone with CT-scan confirmation of complete evacuation of the pleural space or a minimally invasive approach to the incompletely drained space without decortication. Of note is the description of similar re-expansion rates of trapped lung when comparing thorough pleural debridement without decortication with standard open decortication.[11] Further research is needed to arrive at more definitive conclusions. However, this observational study provides further patient-centric decision-making options that should be considered when managing such a challenging patient population. Hofmann and colleagues[12] described their experience with an abbreviated thoracic window and the use of the vacuum-assisted closure (VAC) device for which a limited thoracotomy was made at the site of the empyema followed by the placement of a soft tissue retractor (ALEXIS soft tissue retractor, Applied Medical, Rancho Santa Margarita, CA). A VAC sponge and device were then placed in the pleural space and replaced every 2 to 3 days with good results within 10 days. This process obviated a formal Eloesser flap with its associated morbidity and allowed the patient to resume chemotherapy 1 week after closing the incision, which was achieved with simple stitches.

Pulmonary Resection and Decortication

Patients who have been diagnosed and staged with an obstructing lung cancer without local spread to mediastinal nodes or the pleural space pose a singular challenge. As mentioned earlier in this article, a thorough tissue-proven investigation is mandatory in this group of patients. An empyema and trapped lung complicate the picture by resulting in lymphadenopathy and trapped lung, all of which can be reactive. In the author and colleagues' practice, they proceed with standard mediastinal staging, most commonly with endobronchial ultrasound (EBUS). In this setting, EBUS is a reasonable modality given the lymphadenopathy, which makes for more straightforward targets. Mediastinoscopy is reserved for patients on a case-by-case basis often as the result of a multidisciplinary discussion.

Definitive surgical therapy in this patient population requires a major pulmonary resection in the setting of an infected operative field. All efforts are placed into controlling the infected pleural space locally with appropriate drainage and systemically with antibiotic therapy based on culture results. Once the infectious source has been controlled and preoperative optimization has been achieved, patients should undergo a pulmonary resection, decortication of the remaining lobes, and reinforcement of the bronchial stump. An open approach is necessary given the complexities of the multiple steps required to complete the resection, including procurement of a pedicled muscle flap, adhesiolysis with decortication, and a hilum dissection, which is often hostile. Even though the lobar bronchus to be transected may not be actively infected, the pleural space surrounding it is at risk of developing a postoperative infection that places the stump at risk. Other muscle flaps, such as latissimus dorsi and anterior serratus, are excellent options, particularly when a pleural space is expected in the most challenging cases.

Pain Control Strategy

Complications from thoracic operations are often related to pain that inhibits deep breathing, coughing, and ambulation. Adequate pain control should be a priority within the treatment algorithm of thoracic surgical patients. Despite the increasing use of minimally invasive techniques, pain management requires special attention and, most often, a strategy that involves several techniques. An epidural catheter is a common technique that decreases the use of narcotics. This approach has been proven safe, including in the older population.[13] However, epidural analgesia does not come without potential complications, such as urinary retention, mild hypotension, and epidural hematomas or infection, both of which are reported as rare occurrences. Paraspinal anesthesia has seen an increase in interest with the use of ultrasound guidance and may be a more practical approach to the epidural catheter.[14,15] Local pain control strategies include intercostal nerve block with long-lasting local anesthetic, the placement of a local catheter for continued infusion of analgesic in the subpleural plane, and the use of cryotherapy to induce a temporary neuropraxia, among other techniques. All forms of analgesia, including intravenous and oral medications, have side effects that must be considered in the risks-and-benefits calculations for each patient.

ENDOBRONCHIAL MANAGEMENT OF OBSTRUCTING TUMORS

Bronchoscopy

This article addresses the pleural-space changes that result from endobronchial tumor obstructions and the importance of determining whether those changes are malignancy mediated or a physiologic response to the central bronchial blockage. It is imperative to consider endobronchial measures to relieve the obstruction, which would allow for the improvement of the pleural process while at the same time confirming the diagnosis. Flexible bronchoscopy is commonly the first invasive procedure performed after imaging studies have identified a bronchial obstruction and a pleural effusion. The decision to proceed first with bronchoscopy or thoracentesis should be made on a case-by-case basis, mostly depending on symptoms.

It is important to be prepared at the time of the bronchoscopy to apply several methods and energy sources to treat the obstructed bronchus. Multiple biopsies should be obtained initially, followed by debridement of the bronchus often with an energy source that offers hemostasis. Laser therapy is a well-established method to debulk the tumor. There are several types of lasers in use for this purpose offering different levels of penetration and hemostasis. The review of lasers and bronchoscopy is beyond the scope of this article but is an essential element in the management of these patients. The downsides to laser therapy include the need to reduce the fraction of inspired oxygen (FiO_2) to less than 30%, which may be challenging in patients who present with a large pleural process in addition to the obstruction. In this regard, rigid bronchoscopy affords additional access to the tumor site so that several instruments can be used simultaneously while jet ventilation is used, allowing patients to tolerate lower FiO_2 levels throughout the procedure.

Once the bronchus is patent, patients should undergo a through staging process as described earlier in this text and risk stratified for potential pulmonary resection. The standard approach applies in this situation with the caveat that lung function tests require particular considerations, as patients often present a physiology that has adapted to the loss of function of the involved lobe. Although not ordered routinely in the author's practice, a V/Q scan can be particularly helpful in this situation to allow a more precise interpretation of lung function tests. The ideal time to proceed with resection after bronchoscopic debulking of the obstructing cancer is determined on a case-by-case basis. Proper infection control, cancer staging, and risk stratification are fundamental elements in the decision of when to operate. As mentioned earlier, an open approach with stump buttressing is highly recommended to decrease the possibilities of a bronchopleural fistula (BPF).

SUMMARY

A pleural effusion on the same side of a bronchial cancer is a particular challenge that requires a patient-centered strategy. The management plan should include the treatment of both bronchial obstruction as well as pleural collection in the order that best benefits the individual patient. It is essential that the pleural collection be fully investigated even if asymptomatic, rather than declaring it malignant without tissue confirmation. The level of invasiveness should also be tailored to the situation from a simple thoracentesis to a decortication via thoracotomy. Patients with early stage disease should undergo definitive resection in conjunction with the management of the pleural space, often requiring a combined pulmonary resection and decortication of the remaining lung. It is highly recommended that tissue buttressing of the bronchial stump be offered to decrease the possibilities of BPF. Patients who are not surgical candidates for pulmonary resection but present with an empyema and trapped lung should be considered for one of several alternatives to manage the situation on a case-by-case basis. Tracheobronchial intervention ranges from flexible bronchoscopy under sedation to rigid bronchoscopy under general anesthesia. The goal is to establish the diagnosis, assess the bronchial situation for potential resection, and, where needed, debulking of the endobronchial tumor. Antibiotic therapy and risk stratification will help determine the ideal time for the pulmonary resection to take place.

REFERENCES

1. Miserocchi G. Physiology and pathophysiology of pleural fluid turnover. Eur Respir J 1997;10(1):219–25.
2. Heffner JE, Klein JS. Recent advances in the diagnosis and management of malignant pleural effusions. Mayo Clin Proc 2008;83:235–50.

3. Heffner JE, Nietert PJ, Barbieri C. Pleural fluid pH as a predictor of survival for patients with malignant pleural effusions. Chest 2000;117:79–86.
4. American Thoracic Society. Management of malignant pleural effusions. Am J Respir Crit Care Med 2000;162(5):1987–2001.
5. Thampy E, Cherian SV. The unexpandable lung. N Z Med J 2017;130(1449):64–6.
6. Tattersall DJ, Traill ZC, Gleeson FV. Chest drains: does size matter? Clin Radiol 2000;55:415–21.
7. Rahman NM, Maskell NA, West A, et al. Intrapleural use of tissue plasminogen activator and DNase in pleural Infection. N Engl J Med 2011; 365:518–26.
8. Fysh ET, Tremblay A, Feller-Kopman D, et al. Clinical outcomes of indwelling pleural catheter-related pleural infections: an international multicenter study. Chest 2013;144:1597.
9. Tremblay A, Mason C, Michaud G. Use of tunnelled catheters for malignant pleural effusions in patients fit for pleurodesis. Eur Respir J 2007;30:759–62.
10. Elsayed HH, Hassaballa A, Ahmed T. Is video-assisted thoracoscopic surgery talc pleurodesis superior to talc pleurodesis via tube thoracostomy in patients with secondary spontaneous pneumothorax? Interact Cardiovasc Thorac Surg 2016; 23(3):459–61.
11. Kho P, Karunanantham J, Leung M, et al. Debridement alone without decortication can achieve lung re-expansion in patients with empyema: an observational study. Interact Cardiovasc Thorac Surg 2011; 12(5):724–7.
12. Hofmann HS, Schemm R, Grosser C, et al. Vacuum-assisted closure of pleural empyema without classic open-window thoracostomy. Ann Thorac Surg 2012; 93(5):1741–2.
13. Engelhardt KE, Starnes SL, Hanseman DJ, et al. Epidural versus subpleural analgesia for pulmonary resections: a comparison of morbidities. Am Surg 2014;80(2):109–16.
14. Davies RG, Myles PS, Graham JM. A comparison of the analgesic efficacy and side-effects of paravertebral vs epidural blockade for thoracotomy–a systematic review and meta-analysis of randomized trials. Br J Anaesth 2006;96(4):418–26.
15. Joshi GP, Bonnet F, Shah R, et al. A systematic review of randomized trials evaluating regional techniques for postthoracotomy analgesia. Anesth Analg 2008;107(3):1026–40.

Synchronous Esophageal and Lung Cancer

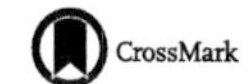

Amar N. Mukerji, MD[a], Andrea Wolf, MD, MPH[b,*]

KEYWORDS

• Lung cancer • Esophageal cancer • Synchronous • Metachronous

KEY POINTS

- Patients with synchronous lung and esophageal cancers must be recognized as having separate cancers rather than metastatic disease of one or the other.
- Each cancer must be staged appropriately and if both are resectable, simultaneous resection may be considered.
- Staged surgical resection and/or surgery in combination with nonoperative therapy (including chemotherapy and/or radiation) may be appropriate.
- Radical resection for noncurative intent (eg, partial resection) should not be performed because this is associated with unacceptable mortality.

INTRODUCTION

Although not a frequently encountered pattern in clinical practice, the care of a patient with concomitant esophageal and lung cancers is a special circumstance, but has been described in the literature.[1–5] Pulmonary and esophageal resection for cancer may carry significant morbidity. When combined, in addition to the technical challenge of the resections themselves, the morbidity of the combined procedures is increased several-fold. When performed in staged fashion in a patient with metachronous tumors, prior treatments for the first cancer (eg, radiation for locally advanced esophageal cancer) may impact the morbidity of resection for the second. The incidence and epidemiology of synchronous esophageal and lung cancer support treatment of this as a unique clinical entity. The technical challenges and the singular morbidity and possible mortality associated with managing such cases merit a discussion of combined lung and esophageal cancers as a special case.

PERSPECTIVES: CONCOMITANT LUNG AND ESOPHAGEAL CARCINOMA IN THE LITERATURE

Most reports of lung and esophageal cancer were published in the Japanese literature. The presence of multiple synchronous primary cancers in patients diagnosed with esophageal cancer is an established pattern in the Japanese population. Many patients with esophageal squamous cell carcinoma (SCC) were found to have another primary SCC in the head and neck (most common), with lung SCC reported less commonly.[6,7] The incidence has been variously reported between 0.54% and 3.2% of patients with esophageal SCC having an associated primary lung cancer.[2,3] The mechanisms of association are not entirely clear but several studies have suggested shared risk factors as a cause insight.[8] Although shared etiologic factors, such as smoking, may predispose patients to both lung and esophageal cancer, the incidence is particularly low. Fekete and coauthors[2] suggested that this may be caused by the

Funding: This work was supported by internal departmental funding.
Conflict of Interest: The authors have no conflict of interest to disclose.
[a] Department of Surgery, Bronx Lebanon Hospital Center, 1650 Selwyn Avenue, Suite 4A, New York, NY 10457, USA; [b] Department of Thoracic Surgery, The Icahn School of Medicine at Mount Sinai, 1190 Fifth Avenue, Box 1022, New York, NY 10029, USA
* Corresponding author.
E-mail address: andrea.wolf@mountsinai.org

Thorac Surg Clin 28 (2018) 97–104
https://doi.org/10.1016/j.thorsurg.2017.09.002

poor prognosis of either cancer, leading to patient death before the second primary can manifest. Alternatively, patients diagnosed with esophageal cancer first (and found to have a lung malignancy) may be misdiagnosed as metastatic (and may be incorrectly staged and treated for either tumor). In most of the reports involving metachronous lung and esophageal cancers, the lung cancer presented first.[2,3,9–11] In most of these reports, lung cancer was treated by radiation. Patients with lung cancer treated with radiation have a relative risk of four to seven of developing a second cancer compared with age-matched normal population.[12,13] Radiation-induced esophageal carcinoma was reported to occur 2 to 19 years following irradiation for breast cancer.[13] More recent reports of metachronous lung followed by esophageal cancers after irradiation for the lung cancer documented an interval of 11 months to 13 years.[3,9] Radiation-induced esophageal cancers after other primary cancer behave differently, perhaps because of differences in risk factors compared with standard esophageal cancer.[12] As such, patients have prominent mediastinal fibrosis and the incidence of lymph node metastasis is lower in radiation-induced esophageal cancers, although survival is equivalent to that of sporadic esophageal malignancies.[2]

SYNCHRONOUS ESOPHAGEAL AND LUNG CANCERS: SPECIAL CONSIDERATIONS

Need for Accurate Diagnosis and Staging

As described by Fekete and coauthors,[2] differentiating between a second primary lung cancer and a lung metastasis from an esophageal cancer in the presence of a synchronous esophageal primary is challenging. Lindenmann and coworkers[14] illustrated the need for accurate staging in a case report of a patient with a midesophageal SCC accompanied by two lung masses. The lung masses were erroneously diagnosed as metastases from the esophagus, but later fortuitously discovered to be synchronous primaries, portending a better prognosis. Lung resection for each with curative intent rather than chemotherapy was the treatment of choice.[14] Although synchronous lung and esophageal cancers are rare in clinical practice, they do occur and clinicians must distinguish double cancers from metastases to determine prognosis and treatment strategies. This should be supported by tissue diagnosis, as illustrated in the report by Lindenmann and coworkers.[14] Suggested criteria that support the diagnosis of primary lung carcinoma are lung tumor with different histology, presence of lung tumor before esophageal carcinoma, solitary lung SCC with endobronchial involvement, or a lung SCC with radiographic appearance of an irregular border/speculation.[2,3,7] Needle biopsy may be useful to obtain tissue diagnosis of the lung lesion, particularly in centers with experienced interventional radiologists and cytopathologists. There are some disadvantages, however, such as risk of pneumothorax, or more uncommonly, hemothorax, and possible nondiagnostic biopsy. Thus, surgical wedge resection is sometimes needed for biopsy. Even minimally invasive video-assisted thoracoscopic surgery (VATS) or robotic-assisted thoracoscopic surgery (RATS) resection may portend risks, including adhesion or complication for definitive esophageal and/or lung resection. These risks should be considered when determining strategy for staging and diagnosis.

Preoperative Risk Assessment: Eligibility for Surgical Treatment of Synchronous Lung and Esophageal Cancer

Although anastomotic or conduit leak represents the most dreaded complication of esophagectomy, other causes of morbidity and mortality for esophagectomy or pulmonary resection include delayed gastric emptying, vocal cord paralysis, airway injury, atrial fibrillation, respiratory failure, pulmonary embolism, myocardial infarction, prolonged air-leak, torsion, and cerebrovascular accident.[15–19] Concomitant surgery for synchronous lung and esophageal cancer may precipitate unexpected mobility of the gastric conduit or the middle lobe (because of extensive disruption of the pulmonary ligament). Given increased risk of complication with combined surgery, meticulous preoperative assessment for suitability for surgery cannot be overemphasized.[18,19] Preoperative assessment should focus on risk-stratifying patients for complex thoracic surgery, with evaluation for inducible myocardial ischemia, ventricular and valvular function, blood gas, spirometry, and quantitative ventilation/perfusion scan as the main components as appropriate. Matsubara and coworkers[18] suggested the following criteria, which have been cited by others.[3,19] Ideal patients should have normal P_{O_2}, normal P_{CO_2}, a forced expiratory volume at 1 second (FEV_1) greater than 70% of vital capacity, and a predicted postoperative vital capacity greater than 50% of the standard value.[18] Shien and coworkers[5] suggested a predicted postoperative FEV_1% (ppo-FEV_1%) greater than 40%. This was calculated by the standard method for pulmonary resection: ppo-FEV_1 = preoperative predicted $FEV_1 \times (19-S)/19$, where S represents the number of bronchopulmonary segments to remove, and 19 represents the total number of bronchopulmonary segments in both lungs.[20] Exceptions were made in carefully selected cases, such as when the lung segments being removed were thought to contribute little to pulmonary function based on size, perfusion, or involvement with tumor.[5,18] Matsubara and coworkers[18] described one patient with extensive bronchiectasis who had an FEV_1 of 65% predicted, but still underwent concomitant esophagectomy and left lower lobectomy because pulmonary perfusion scintigraphy showed minimal pulmonary blood flow through the lobe planned for resection. Similarly, Shien and coworkers[5] described a patient who underwent pulmonary rehabilitation with tiotropium for 3 months to improve ppo-FEV_1% from 36% to 45%.[5]

Operative Planning: Single-Stage Versus Two-Stage Esophageal Reconstruction

Whether to perform resection concomitantly in the case of synchronous lung and esophageal cancers has been discussed and single- versus two-stage surgery has demonstrated comparable rates of complications.[1,2]

Single-stage surgery for resectable synchronous lung and esophageal cancer was reported by several authors.[2,8,18,19,21,22] Several series reported no major postoperative complications.[8,21,22] In other series describing only cases of single-stage surgeries performed with curative intent, significant complications occurred in 20% to 50% of patients, although there were no postoperative deaths.[2,18,19] One study described two deaths in patients who underwent exploratory surgery and complete resections of both cancers were not performed.[2] One death occurred in a patient in whom resection was aborted because of unexpected tracheal involvement of an esophageal tumor. The other death was of a patient who underwent pneumonectomy with a positive bronchial margin, in whom the esophagectomy was not performed because of lack of complete lung cancer resection.

In cases of marginal surgical candidates, some have described a two-staged approach to synchronous lung and esophageal cancer to minimize risk of major pulmonary complication and/or anastomotic leak by performing the resection entirely separately from the restoration of gastrointestinal continuity.[1–3] In the first stage, esophagectomy, lymph node dissection, and pulmonary resection are performed and a temporary cervical esophagostomy is created. Three weeks later, a gastric conduit was mobilized substernally to restore gastrointestinal continuity, thereby separating the risk of anastomotic leak from other complications associated with resection. This method was thought to increase surgical eligibility for high-risk patients with synchronous lung and esophageal cancers. Ishii and coworkers[3] used a two-stage operative strategy because of "fair general condition." A 59-year-old man with a synchronous stage IIA (cT3N0M0) lower thoracic esophageal SCC and a stage IB (cT2N0M0) right segment six adenocarcinoma underwent esophagectomy, cervical esophagostomy, and mediastinal lymph node dissection along with segmentectomy of right pulmonary segment six. Three weeks later a substernal gastric conduit was constructed and the neck and abdominal lymph node dissections were completed. He received chemotherapy with 5-fluorouracil and cisplatin. The authors reported only a wound infection of the neck as postoperative complication and the patient was alive for 10 months with no metastasis at the time of their publication.[3] Other authors have also reported an interval of 3 months. However, in this case, the esophageal cancer was diagnosed after the surgery for lung cancer during evaluation for dysphagia appearing after the lung surgery.[1]

Operative Planning: Incision, Extent of Pulmonary Resection, and Buttressing Bronchial Stump

Given the higher risk of complication with concomitant resection for esophageal and lung cancer, minimizing morbidity is achieved with specific surgical techniques. For example, when approaching via thoracotomy, use of muscle-sparing incision is thought to be better tolerated. VATS or RATS offer even less invasive alternatives. In the short term, thoracotomy results in decreased respiratory excursion and restrictive pulmonary physiology mostly because of splinting. Minimizing the impact of pain and these associated effects is critical and therefore the thoracotomy should be done on the side of the lung lesion, if possible.[2,16,18] There are three main anatomic considerations when planning the incisions: (1) access to the lung tumor, (2) exposure for esophageal mobilization with appropriate lymph node dissection, and (3) adequate access for safe esophageal anastomosis. Approaching both resections from the side of the lung tumor allows access to it. A right-sided approach is usually adequate for esophageal mobilization, lymphadenectomy, and anastomosis. A left-sided approach (eg, thoracoabdominal) may require an additional cervical incision for superior mediastinal esophagogastric anastomosis because of the location of the arch of aorta.[2] Access for lymph node dissection is

Table 1
Literature review

Author	N	Age (y)	Sex	Synchronous or Metachronous	First Cancer if M	Interval if M	Esophageal *Ca Histology*	Esophageal *Ca Location*	Esophageal Ca Stage	Lung Ca Histology	Lung Ca *Location*	Lung Ca *Stage*	Recurrence/ *Survival*	Remarks
Okazaki et al,[9] 1988 (Japanese)	1	61	Male = 1	M	LC	13 y	SCC	Thoracic	—	SCC	RLL	—	Mortality after 7 mo	Both LC and EC treated with definitive radiotherapy Death from pneumonia
Fukuda et al,[21] 1990 (Japanese)	1	69	Male = 1	S	—	—	SCC	Midthoracic	—	SCC	RUL	—	—	—
Morimoto et al,[1] 1991 (Japanese)	2	74 and 66	Male = 2	S	—	—	SCC	Midthoracic, ?	—	Adenoca	LUL	—	74-y patient alive until 22-mo follow-up 66-y patient alive until 18-mo follow-up	The 66-y patient was initially treated as lung metastasis and later diagnosed as histologically distinct
Fékété,[2] 1994	39	Mean 58 (range, 46–68)	Male = 38 Female = 1	S = 22 (58%) M = 17 (44%)	EC = 10 LC = 7	46 mo (18–77 mo)	All SCC	Thoracic = 32 Cervical = 7	I = 7 II = 10 III = 9 NA = 13	SCC = 33 Adenoca = 4 Small cell Ca = 2	Lobar = 27 Bilobar = 5 Lung = 7	I = 17 II = 6 III = 1 NA = 15	Synchronous: 12 with curative surgery, 5-y survival = 11% 2 with palliative surgery died	Synchronous: 14 operative (12 curative 1 stage surgery, 2 palliative surgery); 8 nonoperative (3 radiation, 1 CRT, 4 palliative stenting)
Ishii et al,[3] 2008	4	Mean 62.5 (range, 55–69)	Male = 4	3 S:1 M	LC	11 mo	SCC = 4	Midthoracic = 3 Lower thoracic = 1	I = 1 IIA = 2 III = 1	SCC = 2 Adenoca = 2	RUL = 2 RLL = 1 LLL = 1	IA = 1 IB = 1 IIA = 1 IIB = 1	Variable follow-up of 10–34 mo; all patients alive	Multimodal treatment, including 2-stage definitive surgery (esophageal and lung resection)
Tokumitsu et al,[11] 2009 (Japanese)	1	70	Male = 1	M	LC	5 y	—	Thoracic	II	NSCLC	RUL	IIIB	EC rec Mortality 11 mo after EC diagnosis	LC = CRT, then RUL lobectomy and mediastinal LND EC = Neoadj Chemotherapy, then mediastinoscope assisted transhiatal esophagectomy Postoperative HPE margin positive

Li et al,[4] 2011 (Chinese)	16	Mean 67 (range, 51–76)	Male = 12 Female = 4	S	—	—	—	—	—	—	—	—	87.5% 1-y survival	—
Shien et al,[5] 2011	6	Median 75 (range, 69–80)	Male = 5 Female = 1	M = 5 S = 1	EC = 5	25 mo (3–71 mo)	SCC	Upper thoracic = 3 Lower thoracic = 3	Stage II = 2 Stage III = 4	SCC = 4 Adenoca = 2	RUL = 2 RLL = 1 LUL = 2 LLL = 1	Stage IA = 6	Variable length of follow-up median 25 mo (range, 13–73 mo) EC recurrence = 2; alive = 4	EC = all 6 CRT, salvage surgery in 1 LC = 4 segmentectomy, 2 lobectomy 5 had mediastinal LND, 5 VATS, 1 open
Wang et al,[19] 2012	14	Mean 60.7 (range, 49–76)	Male = 14	S = 6 EC invading lung = 8	—	—	SCC = 12 Adenoca = 2	Midthoracic = 5 Lower thoracic = 7 Cardia = 2	—	SCC = 1 Adenoca = 4 Tuberculosis = 1 Tracheoesophageal fistula = 1	RUL = 2 RLL = 1 LUL = 1 LLL = 2	—	Variable follow-up of 1–90 mo; 6 of 14 patients alive Six deaths caused by metastases, 1 local recurrence, 1 postoperative death	Only 1 death immediate postoperative death caused by cardiopulmonary issues Mean hospital stay = 17 d (range, 7–30 d) 4/14 (30.8%) postoperative complication rate
Song et al,[8] 2016	1	63	Female = 1	S	—	—	SCC	Midthoracic	IIA	Adenoca	—	IA	No recurrence after 6 mo of follow-up	Synchronous esophageal + lung + thymoma (type AB, stage I) Concurrent (in the sequence below) 1. VATS thymectomy 2. VATS RUL lobectomy + LND 3. Video-assisted thoracolaparoscopic esophagectomy + 2 field LND

Abbreviations: Adenoca, adenocarcinoma; Ca, cancer; CRT, chemoradiotherapy; EC, esophageal cancer; HPE, histopathologic examination; LC, lung cancer; LLL, left lower lobe; LND, lymph node dissection; LUL, left upper lobe; M, metachronous; NSCLC, non–small cell lung cancer; RLL, right lower lobe; RUL, right upper lobe; S, synchronous.

particularly challenging. Matsubara and coworkers[18] recommended considering a cervical incision with or without median sternotomy for complete dissection of superior mediastinal lymph nodes by the recurrent laryngeal nerves, because of their higher propensity of metastatic involvement.[18] Accounting for the lower incidence of lymph node involvement in the vicinity of the aortic arch, a less extensive lymphadenectomy may be tolerated in this area.

The extent of pulmonary resection impacts short- and long-term outcomes. Pneumonectomy was associated with high risk of mortality, and thus Fekete cautioned against performing concurrent pneumonectomy with esophagectomy.[2,23] It is likely that the dissection near the airway (with possible skeletonization of the bronchial stump) and a fresh esophagogastric anastomosis in a pneumonectomy space may increase the risk of empyema and/or bronchopleural fistula. Most reports described more acceptable morbidity and mortality in the setting of concomitant lobectomy and esophagectomy.

Reinforcement of the bronchial stump with a vascularized tissue flap in the setting of an anatomic lung resection when performed with esophagectomy is advised. Choices are restricted in the setting of prior radiation and/or surgery, however. Various techniques have been described and the choice for a given case needs to be tailored individually, avoiding harvesting a flap from tissues in a previously irradiated field. Options include intercostal muscle flap, latissimus dorsi flap, pericardial flap, anterior mediastinal fat flap, and omental flap from the gastric conduit. Minimally invasive approaches to a combined esophagectomy lung resection (and, in one case report of concomitant thymoma, thymectomy) have been described.[8,22] The advantage of minimally invasive approach with VATS or RATS is that bilateral surgery may be better tolerated and therefore right- and left-sided approaches may allow better anatomic access.[8]

A Comment on Metachronous Cancers

Surgery for a metachronous tumor in the setting of prior resection (lung if prior esophagectomy, or esophagectomy if prior pulmonary resection) is by definition reoperative. This results in higher risk of complication, because the chest or the mediastinum has already been exposed to previous surgery and, sometimes, radiation.

SYSTEMATIC REVIEW OF THE LITERATURE

A systematic review of the literature was performed via PubMed using the following search terms: ((“lung cancer”[ti/abstract] OR “lung carcinoma”[ti/abstract]) AND (“esophageal cancer”[ti/abstract] OR “esophageal carcinoma”[ti/abstract])) AND (“concomitant”[tw] OR “simultaneous”[tw] OR “concurrent”[tw] OR “synchronous”[tw] OR “together”[tw] OR “metachronous”[tw] OR “second primary”[tw] OR “multiple primary”[tw] OR “double cancer”[tw]). These articles were read individually and their bibliographies were searched with relevant reports included as a secondary search. Articles in other languages with English abstracts also were considered (**Table 1**). The literature regarding simultaneous lung and esophageal cancer is sparse. Most reports were from Japan. The largest series, which included both synchronous and metachronous lesions, was a French series published by Fekete and coworkers.[2] Matsubara and colleagues[18] published their extensive experience focusing on esophageal and pulmonary surgery either simultaneously or sequentially. This series described surgical and perioperative issues for patients undergoing lung and esophageal surgery, for benign and malignant disease. Most patients were in their 50s to 60s (range, 46–80). Most were male (62 of 69; 89.9%), with SCC as the histology for all esophageal tumors and most (42 of 60; 70%) lung tumors.[2,3,5,9,19,21] Most of the remaining lung tumors were adenocarcinoma (12 of 60; 90%).[1–3,5,8,19] Fifty-two out of the 77 cancer concomitant patients (67.5%) had synchronous tumors, and 25 (32.5%) had metachronous tumors. Most patients with synchronous cancers underwent single-stage surgery. Ishii and coworkers[3] recommended a two-stage procedure to avoid pulmonary complications and an anastomotic leak at the same time, with the goal of increasing surgical candidacy for marginal patients. Recent reports recommended minimally invasive approaches.[8,22]

Nonsurgical treatment options have also been described as adjuncts to surgery or as primary therapy. Among the 12 patients in this series who underwent curative surgery, two received preoperative chemoradiotherapy for suspected mediastinal involvement, and one received chemoradiation postoperatively because the lung tumor was small cell cancer. The 5-year survival of the 12 patients treated with curative intent was 11%.[2] Ishii and coworkers[3] reported using primary chemoradiation based on 5-fluorouracil and cisplatin for two patients with synchronous tumors with obstructive respiratory disease and deemed unfit for surgery. They reported a 28 and 34 months of disease-free follow-up.[3] Most authors have used surgery as the primary therapy with chemotherapy and radiations as adjuncts. However, they are viable options in case of unresectable lesions or in patients who are otherwise poor surgical candidates.

With a follow-up of 6 to 87 months for all studies, major postoperative complications were rarely seen, but no immediate postoperative mortality occurred in patients undergoing surgery with curative intent. There were two deaths and these were in the setting of palliative surgery and a combined pneumonectomy/esophagectomy. In the largest series, Fekete and coworkers[2] reported a 5-year survival of 11% for patients with synchronous lung and esophageal cancer treated with curative surgery.[2]

In patients with metachronous cancers who presented with esophageal cancer first, the subsequent lung cancers were diagnosed by surveillance computed tomography (CT), and were therefore mostly diagnosed at an early stage. In contrast, in patients with metachronous cancers who presented with lung cancer first, the esophageal malignancies were diagnosed at a later stage because CT is less sensitive for early mucosal lesions. Although the incidence of metachronous lung and esophageal cancer was too low to recommend a screening regimen, early investigation with esophagram and/or enodoscopy should be considered for symptoms and/or CT abnormalities in the esophagus.[2,3] A full discussion on metachronous cancers is beyond the scope of this article.

SUMMARY

Concomitant lung and esophageal cancer is a known clinical entity, although it is rare and sparsely reported in literature. Most patients are men in their 50s to 60s. The histology for the esophageal cancer is almost always SCC, and the lung cancer is more often SCC. Synchronous cancers are often confused for metastases, and therefore a meticulous diagnostic work-up should consider the possibility of concomitant cancers. If both tumors are resectable, preoperative pulmonary risk assessment includes blood gas, FEV_1, and ppo-FEV_1. Surgery is performed in one or two stages, with the latter intended to minimize concomitant major postoperative morbidity and mortality. The literature suggests a benefit to curative surgery, but aggressive surgery with palliative intent has been associated with unacceptable mortality risk. When planning surgery for synchronous tumors, the incisions should be placed on the side of the lung lesion, and additional access is obtained by a cervical incision or contralateral VATS/RATS, depending on approach. For thoracotomy, a muscle-sparing incision is preferable and minimally invasive approaches are considered. Simultaneous lobectomy or sublobar resection has been safely performed with esophagectomy, but patient selection for concomitant pneumonectomy with esophagectomy should be considered carefully because the risk of mortality may be prohibitive. Although long-term survival for patients with concomitant lung and esophageal cancer is low compared with those with either one or the other, the survival with curative surgery is higher than that of patients with metastatic disease of either primary. Nonoperative therapies, such as definitive chemoradiation for esophageal or lung cancer, and stereotactic radiation for lung cancer, should be considered in patients who cannot tolerate one or both resections. Careful evaluation of patients presenting with suspicious esophageal and lung lesions should be performed to investigate the possibility of concomitant primaries and tailor the therapeutic strategy to optimize patient outcomes.

REFERENCES

1. Morimoto M, Ohno T, Yamashita Y, et al. Two surgical cases of synchronous double carcinoma of the lung and esophagus and review of 10 documented cases in Japan. Nihon Kyobu Geka Gekkai Zasshi 1991; 39(2):245–50 [in Japanese].
2. Fékété F, Sauvanet A, Kaisserian G, et al. Associated primary esophageal and lung carcinoma: a study of 39 patients. Ann Thorac Surg 1994;58(3): 837–42.
3. Ishii H, Sato H, Tsubosa Y, et al. Treatment of double carcinoma of the esophagus and lung. Gen Thorac Cardiovasc Surg 2008;56(3):126–30.
4. Li F, Shao K, Xue Q, et al. Clinical observation of 16 patients with synchronous esophageal cancer and lung cancer treated with simultaneous esophagus and lung resection. Zhonghua Yi Xue Za Zhi 2011; 91(15):1064–6 [in Chinese].
5. Shien K, Yamashita M, Okazaki M, et al. Primary lung cancer surgery after curative chemoradiotherapy for esophageal cancer patients. Interact Cardiovasc Thorac Surg 2011;12(6):1002–6.
6. Vyas JJ, Deshpande RK, Sharma S, et al. Multiple primary cancers in Indian population: metachronous and synchronous lesions. J Surg Oncol 1983;23(4): 239–49.
7. Imada T, Sato H, Hasuo K, et al. Development of synchronous bilateral lung cancers after esophagectomy for esophageal cancer: report of a case. Surg Today 1998;28(10):1042–5.
8. Song X, Shen H, Li J, et al. Minimally invasive resection of synchronous triple primary tumors of the esophagus, lung, and thymus: a case report. Int J Surg Case Rep 2016;29:59–62.

9. Okazaki A, Matsuura M, Noda M, et al. Esophageal cancer developing 13 years after radiotherapy of lung cancer. Gan No Rinsho 1988;34(6):787–93 [in Japanese].
10. Otsuka Y, Konishi T, Nara S, et al. Secondary myelodysplastic syndrome after small cell lung cancer and esophageal cancer. J Gastroenterol Hepatol 2005;20(9):1318–21.
11. Tokumitsu Y, Yamamoto T, Kitamura Y, et al. A case of mediastinoscope-assisted transhiatal esophagectomy for thoracic esophageal cancer after radical operation for lung cancer. Gan To Kagaku Ryoho 2009;36(12):2445–7 [in Japanese].
12. Goffman TE, McKeen EA, Curtis RE, et al. Esophageal carcinoma following irradiation for breast cancer. Cancer 1983;52(10):1808–9.
13. Ueda M, Matsubara T, Kasumi F, et al. Possible radiation induced cancer of the thoracic esophagus after postoperative irradiation in breast cancer. Nihon Kyobu Geka Gakkai Zasshi 1991;39(10):1852–7 [in Japanese].
14. Lindenmann J, Matzi V, Maier A, et al. Transthoracic esophagectomy and lobectomy performed in a patient with synchronous lung cancer and combined esophageal cancer and esophageal leiomyosarcoma. Eur J Cardiothorac Surg 2007;31(2):322–4.
15. Müller JM, Erasmi H, Stelzner M, et al. Surgical therapy of oesophageal carcinoma. Br J Surg 1990; 77(8):845–57.
16. Nagawa H, Kobori O, Muto T. Prediction of pulmonary complications after transthoracic oesophagectomy. Br J Surg 1994;81(6):860–2.
17. Dumont P, Wihlm JM, Hentz JG, et al. Respiratory complications after surgical treatment of esophageal cancer. A study of 309 patients according to the type of resection. Eur J Cardio-thorac Surg 1995;9(10):539–43.
18. Matsubara T, Ueda M, Takahashi T, et al. Surgical treatment of cancer of the thoracic esophagus in association with a major pulmonary operation. J Am Coll Surg 1997;185(6):520–4.
19. Wang XX, Liu TL, Wang P, et al. Is surgical treatment of cancer of the gastric cardia or esophagus associated with a concurrent major pulmonary operation feasible? One center's experience. Chin Med J (Engl) 2012;125(2):193–6.
20. Kearney DJ, Lee TH, Reilly JJ, et al. Assessment of operative risk in patients undergoing lung resection. Importance of predicted pulmonary function. Chest 1994;105(3):753–9.
21. Fukuda H, Ogino N, Takao T, et al. A case report of synchronous double cancer of the lung and esophagus. Nihon Kyobu Geka Gakkai Zasshi 1990;38(6): 1053–8 [in Japanese].
22. Dolci G, Dell'Amore A, Asadi N, et al. Synchronous thymoma and lung adenocarcinoma treated with a single mini-invasive approach. Heart Lung Circ 2015;24(1):e11–3.
23. Tachimori Y, Watanabe H, Kato H. Left pneumonectomy associated with subtotal esophagectomy for carcinoma of the esophagus invading the left main bronchus. Jpn J Clin Oncol 1989;19(2):167–9.

Thoracic Surgery in Patients with AIDS

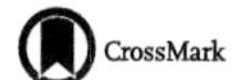

Doraid Jarrar, MD*, Grace Y. Song, MD

KEYWORDS

• HIV • AIDS • Thoracic surgery

KEY POINTS

- Thoracic surgery had its origin for the treatment of infections of the pleural space, mostly related to complications of tuberculosis.
- Human immunodeficiency virus infection and AIDS are a spectrum of conditions caused by infections with the human deficiency virus.
- As the infection progresses, it compromises the immune system, increasing the risk of common infections like tuberculosis as well as other opportunistic infections and also giving rise to tumors.
- Specifically, infections, such as pneumocystis pneumonia and esophageal candidiasis, may require the attention of a thoracic surgeon.

INTRODUCTION

Thoracic surgery had its origin for the treatment of infections of the pleural space, mostly related to complications of tuberculosis (TB). Human immunodeficiency virus (HIV) infection and AIDS are a spectrum of conditions caused by infections with the human deficiency virus. As the infection progresses, it compromises the immune system, increasing the risk of common infections like TB as well as other opportunistic infections and also giving rise to tumors. Specifically, infections, such as pneumocystis pneumonia and esophageal candidiasis, may require the attention of a thoracic surgeon. In this article, the authors discuss the care of patients with HIV as it pertains to thoracic surgery and how these patients may present with different issues than non-HIV patients.

PNEUMOTHORAX

Pneumothoraxes are uncommon in HIV-infected patients but could portend an overall poor prognosis.[1] The causes of pneumothoraxes in those patients are many, including Kaposi sarcoma, toxoplasmosis, bacterial, fungal, and viral and mycobacterial infections; but most often it is pneumocystis jiroveci pneumonia (PCP).[2] The possible risk factors are aerosolized pentamidine, low CD4 count, cigarette smoking, and PCP infection. The treatment is similar to non–HIV-infected patients, with observation of small pneumothoraxes and chest tube thoracostomy for larger pneumothoraxes or tension physiology. Although this would be categorized as a secondary pneumothorax, immediate surgical intervention is not obligatory. The same principles as for primary spontaneous pneumothoraxes can be applied, with the lowest recurrence rate being reported for thoracotomy and pleurectomy but very high success rates also with video-assisted thoracoscopic surgery, pleural abrasion, or partial pleurectomy. Chemical pleurodesis is also a choice, although the authors reserve those for malignant effusions.[3]

Disclosures: The authors disclose no potential conflicts of interest.
Division of Thoracic Surgery, Perelman School of Medicine at the University of Pennsylvania, Penn Presbyterian Medical Center, 51 North 39th Street, WS Suite 266, Philadelphia, PA 19141, USA
* Corresponding author.
E-mail address: doraidj@yahoo.com

Thorac Surg Clin 28 (2018) 105–108
https://doi.org/10.1016/j.thorsurg.2017.09.005

NECROTIZING ESOPHAGITIS

Necrotizing esophagitis (black esophagus) is a rare, potentially lethal finding that can progress to esophageal perforation. Although very rare, it is more common in patients with AIDS and other hematologic malignancies and carries an extremely high mortality rate, exceeding 50%.[4] As reported by Gaissert and colleagues,[4] mortality without intervention was 90% and is lowest in patients with surgical intervention, 27%. In their series, intervention ranged from stenting and drainage to esophagectomy, with 8 out of 11 patients surviving. It is more common for patients with HIV to have infectious esophagitis, but progression to necrosis is rare.[5] The clinical presentation can be as insidious as hematemesis and melena as well as incidental findings on endoscopy for other reasons to fulminant sepsis because of perforation.

PLEURAL EFFUSION IN PATIENTS WITH HUMAN IMMUNODEFICIENCY VIRUS

Pleural effusions are common among patients with AIDS and in hospitalized patients the prevalence varies up to 27%.[6] Most effusions are caused by infections, but noninfectious causes are found in up to one-third of cases. Opportunistic infections are more frequent with a CD4 count less than 150 cells per microliter. Because viral infections are responsible for some of the malignant effusions (Kaposi's sarcoma [KS], multicentric Castleman disease, primary effusion lymphoma), the distinction between infectious and noninfectious is less clear. Bacterial pneumonia, especially *Streptococcus pneumonia*, is common and can lead to an empyema, requiring thoracic consultation and treatment beyond just simple thoracentesis.[7,8] Pleural effusions due to PCP are uncommon and can also cause pleural masses and pneumothorax.[9] Mycobacterium TB and mycobacterium avium complex account for around 10% of pleural effusions in patients with AIDS. Pleural TB can present without parenchymal disease and only a pleural effusion. The effusion is almost always exudative with normal pH and glucose levels. The nucleated cell count is usually lower than in non-HIV patients with TB pleurisy; the effusion is predominant lymphocytic.[10]

CANCER AND HUMAN IMMUNODEFICIENCY VIRUS

Patients with AIDS have an increased incidence of Kaposi sarcoma (including pulmonary), intermediate- or high-grade lymphoma, and uterine cervical cancer. Kaposi sarcoma is a low-grade vascular tumor associated with human herpesvirus 8 (HHV-8). HHV-8 is also linked to primary effusion lymphoma and multicentric Castleman disease. The incidence of pulmonary Kaposi sarcoma is difficult to determine but was found in 47% of autopsies of patients with cutaneous lesions.[11] The main presenting symptoms are cough and shortness of breath. Hemoptysis can occur, and patients have cutaneous lesions as presented in the study by Miller and colleagues.[12] Pleural effusions are common; in general, pulmonary and pleural involvement is a harbinger of a short life expectancy. Bronchoscopy will usually yield a diagnosis, but lesions can also be found on the visceral and parietal pleura during thoracoscopy. The main treatment of pulmonary KS is antiretroviral therapy (ART), which takes a few months to see an initial spike in CD4 count. Before ART, the outlook was dismal and combination chemotherapy was given, with decent response rates.[13]

Non-Hodgkin lymphoma (NHL) is another AIDS-defining malignancy due to the impaired cellular immunity. Among those with HIV, approximately 10% will develop an NHL, with primary effusion lymphoma being the least common of the acquired AIDS-related lymphomas.[14] These body cavity–based lymphomas represent as lymphoma cells in serosa lined cavities (pleura, pericardium, and peritoneum). There is no tumor mass, lymphadenopathy, or organomegaly. The key diagnostic criterion is the presence of HHV-8 in the nuclei of malignant cells.[15] A chest radiograph shows unilateral or bilateral pleural effusion with no parenchymal infiltrates or mediastinal adenopathy. Computed tomography of the chest usually confirms these findings with slight thickening of the parietal pleura.[16] The differential diagnosis includes systemic lymphomas with secondary involvement of the body fluid and lymphomas that develop as a result of chronic pyothorax. The presence of HHV-8 positivity can help distinguish primary effusion lymphoma from others.[15]

LUNG CANCER AND HUMAN IMMUNODEFICIENCY VIRUS

The deadliest cancer worldwide, lung cancer, has a higher incidence in HIV-infected patients than in the general population.[17,18] Also, HIV-infected patients tended to be younger, the cancer more advanced, and adenocarcinoma the most frequent histologic diagnosis.

The risk of lung cancer is significantly higher in patients with HIV (2–4 fold) and has not changed with the introduction of ART. Even after correcting for smoking status, the risk of lung cancer remains elevated compared with age- and sex-matched non–HIV-infected populations.[18,19] The study by D'Jean and colleagues[20] using the Surveillance Epidemiology and End Results (SEER) program showed that in the era of ART, HIV-related lung cancer diagnosis was at the median age of 50 years, compared with 68 years for SEER participants and, most frequently, like their non–HIV-positive counterparts, presented with stage IIIB/IV disease. Tumor types and survival were similar. These findings are interesting because smoking is usually more prevalent in HIV-positive patients and screening in the appropriate population is not recommended until 55 years of age, as published in the National Lung Screening trial.[21] The French HIV CHEST study team showed that lung cancer screening in patients younger than 55 years is warranted in HIV-positive patients. Their patients had at least a 20 pack-year history, aged 40 years and older, and a nadir CD4+ T-cell count less than 350 cells per microliter, with a current CD4+ T-cell count of at least 100 cells per microliter. Their study included 442 patients; the incidence of lung cancer after 2 years of screening was 2%, with most detected in patients younger than 55 years.[22,23] These studies suggest that one should include lung cancer in the differential diagnosis in infected patients when presenting with pulmonary symptoms, although they may not meet the typical age criteria. A recent study by Coghill and colleagues[24] highlights the excess mortality among HIV-infected individuals with regard to lung cancer, as there are now effective antiviral medications prolonging the life to near-normal life expectancy. This finding suggests that HIV may contribute to cancer progression in ways incompletely understood at this time. Oxidative stress, expression of matrix metalloproteinases, and genetic instability may explain this increased susceptibility and a shift from predominantly infectious complications to noninfectious lung disease.[25]

SUMMARY

The picture of HIV-infected patients has changed dramatically since the original description in 1981. The introduction of antiretroviral drugs in 1987 and combination ART has decreased mortality by as much as 80%. We now see patients in their 60s and 70s, having lived decades with HIV and living a normal live. As outlined in the article, despite good viral control, patients with HIV may present with solid organ cancers earlier than noninfected patients and are also prone to other complications of their disease that may require attention of a thoracic surgeon.

REFERENCES

1. Afessa B. Pleural effusion and pneumothorax and hospitalized patients with HIV infection: the pulmonary complications, ICU support, and prognostic factors of hospitalist patient with HIV (PIP) study. Chest 2000;117:1031–7.
2. Beers MF, Sohn M, Swartz M. Recurrent pneumothorax in AIDS patients with Pneumocystis pneumonia. A clinicopathologic report of three cases and review of the literature. Chest 1990;98:266–70.
3. Kimmel RD, Karp MD, Cascone JJ, et al. Talc pleurodesis during VATS for Pneumocystis carinii pneumonia-related pneumothorax. A new technique. Chest 1994;105:314–5.
4. Gaissert HA, Roper CL, Patterson GA, et al. Infectious necrotizing esophagitis: outcome after medical and surgical intervention. Ann Thorac Surg 2003;75:342–7.
5. Hoffman M, Bash E, Berger SA, et al. Fatal necrotizing esophagitis due to Penicillium chrysogenum in a patient with acquired immunodeficiency syndrome. Eur J Clin Microbiol Infect Dis 1992;11:1158–60.
6. Joseph J, Strange C, Sahn SA. Pleural effusions in hospitalized patients with AIDS. Ann Intern Med 1993;118:856–9.
7. Armbruster C, Schalleschak J, Vetter N, et al. Pleural effusions in human immune-deficiency virus-infected patients. Correlation with concomitant pulmonary disease. Acta Cytol 1995;39:698–700.
8. Gil Suay V, Cordero PJ, Martinez E, et al. Parapneumonic effusions secondary to community-acquired bacterial pneumonia in human immunodeficiency virus-infected patients. Eur Respir J 1995;8:1934–9.
9. Jayes RL, Kamerow HN, Hasselquist SM, et al. Disseminated pneumocystosis presenting as a pleural effusion. Chest 1993;103:306–8.
10. Gopi A, Madhavan SM, Sharma SK, et al. Diagnosis and treatment of tuberculous pleural effusion in 2006. Chest 2007;131:880–9.
11. Meduri GU, Stover DE, Lee M, et al. Pulmonary Kaposi's sarcoma in the acquired immune deficiency syndrome. Clinical, radiographic, and pathologic manifestations. Am J Med 1986;81:11–8.
12. Miller RF, Tomlinson MC, Cottrill CP, et al. Bronchopulmonary Kaposi's sarcoma in patients with AIDS. Thorax 1992;47:721–5.
13. Gill PS, Rarick M, McCutchan JA, et al. Systemic treatment of AIDS-related Kaposi's sarcoma: results of a randomized trial. Am J Med 1991;90:427–33.
14. Simonelli C, Spina M, Cinelli R, et al. Clinical features and outcome of primary effusion lymphoma in HIV-infected patients: a single institution study. J Clin Oncol 2003;21:3948–54.
15. Carbone A, Gloghini A. KSHV/HHV8-associated lymphomas. Br J Haematol 2008;140:13–24.

16. Morassut S, Vaccher E, Balestreri L, et al. HIV-associated human herpesvirus8-positive primary lymphomatous effusions: radiologic findings in six patients. Radiology 1997;205:459–63.
17. Deeken JF, Tjen-A-Looi A, Rudek MAI, et al. The rising challenge of non-AIDS defining cancers in HIV-infected patients. Clin Infect Dis 2012;55:1228–35.
18. Kirk GD, Merlo C, O'Driscoll P, et al. HIV infection is associated with an increased risk for lung cancer, independent of smoking. Clin Infect Dis 2007;45: 103–10.
19. Clifford GM, Lise M, Franceschi S, et al. Lung cancer in the Swiss HIV Cohort Study: role of smoking, immunodeficiency and pulmonary infection. Br J Cancer 2012;106:447–52.
20. D'Jean GA, Pantanowitz L, Bower M, et al. Human immunodeficiency virus-associated primary lung cancer in the area of highly active antiretroviral therapy: a multi-institutional collaboration. Clin Lung Cancer 2010;11:396–404.
21. National Lung Screening Trial Research Team, Aberle DR, Adams AM, et al. Reduced lung-cancer mortality with low-dose computed tomographic screening. N Eng J Med 2011;365:395–409.
22. Bommart S, Cournil A, Eymard-Duvernay S, et al. Smoking-associated morbidities on computed tomography lung cancer screens in HIV-infected smokers. HIV Med 2017;1–5.
23. Makinson A, Eymard-Duvernay S, Raffi F, et al. Feasibility and efficacy of early lung cancer diagnosis with chest computed tomography in HIV infected smokers. AIDS 2016;20:573–82.
24. Coghill AE, Pfeiffer RM, Shiels MS, et al. Excess mortality among HIV-infected individuals with cancer in the United States. Cancer Epidemiol Biomarkers Prev 2017;26:1–7.
25. Presti RM, Flores SC, Palmer BE, et al. Mechanisms underlying HIV associated non-infectious lung disease. Chest 2017. [Epub ahead of print].

Printed and bound by CPI Group (UK) Ltd, Croydon, CR0 4YY
08/05/2025
01864707-0004